What Healthcare Professionals are Saying About *Why We Overeat and How to Stop*

Elizabeth Babcock has written the most helpful and comprehensive book on overeating I have ever seen ... The book is extremely well written and thoroughly referenced. Babcock breaks things down to make them understandable and memorable ...

This book takes the reader by the hand to design a new life without overeating, from the ways to think about such a life (long term well-being, a satisfying life) to the step-by-step practical strategies that lead there ... It is a worthy read for anyone, and a godsend for those who seek to enjoy a satisfying life without overeating.

Sharon Eakes, MA, BCC; Executive Coach, Author, Huffington Post Blogger, Clinical Director (1972-1996) of Gateway Rehabilitation Center, Aliquippa, PA

Ms. Babcock ... offers an easily understood overview of how our brains function in relation to compulsive behaviors such as overeating, explaining how the emotional brain often sabotages our ability to maintain control as it seeks immediate gratification through eating ...

Why We Overeat and How to Stop moves beyond thinking of diets, pounds, numbers, and scales and challenges readers to critically appraise overeating, set meaningful, individualized goals, and move beyond all-or-nothing thinking in an effort to promote our healthiest selves ...

I certainly plan to recommend this book to clients who struggle with eating issues and also feel that this book can benefit anyone struggling with compulsive behaviors.

Kirstyn M. Kameg, DNP, PMHNP-BC; Professor of Nursing, AIME Project Director, PMHNP Program Coordinator; Robert Morris University, School of Nursing & Health Sciences

Babcock ... combines compassion, science-supported information, and a practical guide to light the way toward a sustainable and joyful relationship with food. In doing so, she also points the way for us to create deeply meaningful lives revolving around what matters most ...

She invites us to let ourselves off the hook, and make a life-change for the better. Very rarely do self-help books offer tangible, accessible steps with such clarity and depth of heart.

Dr. Lori Gray, PhD; Licensed Psychologist, Assistant Professor; Integrative Holistic Health and Wellness, Western Michigan University

Elizabeth Babcock has written one of the most easily "digested" self-help books I have ever read. *Why We Overeat and How to Stop* provides a wealth of information about how evolution, neuroscience, culture, and society influence the way we eat, and, more importantly, many well-thought-out and tested strategies for making profound life changes. She manages to convey all of this in a conversational style without jargon or undue complexity. It is as though she is sitting across the room from and talking directly to the reader. Her insight, compassion, and support emanate throughout. *Why We Overeat and How to Stop* is an invaluable resource for people struggling with overeating and the professionals who are trying to help them.

Robert Mason, LCSW CEAP; Director of Employee Assistance Services; 21st Century Employee Assistance Partners, Inc., Pittsburgh, PA

This book is nothing short of remarkable in its ability to address the dynamics of overeating in a clear and understandable manner as well as those processes needed to make change ... I highly recommend this book for individuals who have fought with overeating and for anyone wishing to treat clients who have had any issues around eating. It is easily understood and written in language that can be followed by clients, and novice as well as seasoned clinicians.

Dr. John D Massella, LPC, NCC, CCS, CCDP; Assistant Professor and Clinician, California University of Pennsylvania

In Ms. Babcock's book, *Why We Overeat and How to Stop*, she provides compelling insight into the fundamental reasons why all of us are prone to overeating. The all-encompassing comprehensive approach to this book truly makes it stand out ...

The book is thoroughly researched, well written, and wide reaching. It touches upon the importance of our emotional behaviors (you may think twice about giving your crying baby a snack to calm him down after reading this book), the challenge of the American diet as it currently stands, and the utmost importance in which exercise minimizes overeating.

It has proven to be a very enjoyable read, with practical advice that just makes sense, and I intend to wholeheartedly recommend this book to my patients going forward.

Jeffrey Liu, MD; Clinical Cardiac Electrophysiologist
South Hills Cardiology Associates, Bethel Park, PA

I have followed wellness-related media for decades now, but was pleasantly surprised to find something totally new here ... This material is a complete, near-encyclopedic work aimed at weight-regulating mechanisms of the human body ... Some chapters are very unique and familiar only to highly specialized health professionals ... yet reading them is easy and entertaining.

This book is a game changer. I highly recommend it to the general public as well as to health care providers at all levels.

Evgeniy A. Shchelchkov, MD; Chairman, Department of Neurology; The Washington Health System, Washington, PA

As someone who has battled food addiction all of my life, I find Ms. Babcock's words and concepts so simple that I wonder why no one else has ever been able to fine-tune the art of normalizing food consumption and taking the fight out of the process ...

Her approach to why we eat, how we eat, how we choose our food, how we shop and most certainly what we define as food should be the foundation for the way we honor our bodies and thus feed not only our physical self but our soul.

Debra Bates, RN; Director of Health Ministries
Christ United Methodist Church, Bethel Park, PA

In this practical, readable, intellectually digestible resource, Ms. Babcock explains in simple terms the complex neurobiology of eating and overeating, of cravings, and of one's preference for being a couch potato rather than an Energizer Bunny®. More importantly, Ms. Babcock explains how to work with rather than against nature to improve one's physical well-being, while simultaneously improving one's mental well-being ...

While this book is intended for individuals struggling with emotional food and eating issues, health professionals would certainly benefit from reading it as well. I recommend it for counselors/psychotherapists, Registered Dietitian Nutritionists, personal trainers, health coaches, Registered Nurses, and primary care providers (MDs/DOs/CRNPs/PAs).

Katherine Stephens-Bogard, MS, RDN/LD, CDE, RYT; Registered Dietitian Nutritionist, Certified Diabetes Educator; DEMP & Outpatient Nutrition, The Washington Health System, Washington, PA

Why We Overeat

and

How to Stop

Elizabeth Babcock, LCSW

ELIZABETH A BABCOCK, LCSW, LLC
MCMURRAY, PENNSYLVANIA

WHY WE OVEREAT AND HOW TO STOP
July 2016

Published by:
Elizabeth A. Babcock, LCSW, LLC
4050 Washington Road, Suite 3G
McMurray, PA 15317
www.elizabethbabcock.com
www.facebook.com

Library of Congress Control Number: 2016909251

ISBN-13: 978-1533410290
ISBN-10: 1533410291

Printed in the United States of America
First Edition

To everyone who has ever felt enslaved by food.

Contents

Part Three
Common Psychological Hurdles
on the Path Toward Change

Contents

Part Four
Building a Stronger Base for Your Future

Part Five
Eating with Dignity and Enjoyment for Life

Preface

If you have spent years struggling to keep your overeating under control or if you've given up the fight altogether, this book is for you. Whether or not you are actually overweight, it is the internal torment of overeating that this book is meant to address. I know the struggle personally, having once spent close to four decades there myself.

My overeating started around age five or six, which I've since learned is the most common age for it to begin. By second grade I was clearly becoming "the fat kid," something of an oddity in the 1960s when I grew up. I spent my childhood feeling self-conscious, ashamed, and oddly confused about it all.

My weight kept creeping up relative to my peers, but it wasn't until a memorable time in seventh grade when I gained 14 pounds in 14 days that I realized this was something I needed to try to control. I was able to level off at that new weight and stayed there for over a year—until the crazy dieting started.

I got down to a more normal weight by high school, but only through repeated brute-force diets of my own design which, in retrospect, were remarkably unhealthy. It was the best effort of an adolescent, I suppose. I never, ever ate normally. I just alternated between dieting and the rebound pursuit of salty, fatty, sugary junk food, in cycles that might last days or weeks, but seldom as long as months. To this day, I marvel that I managed to enter adulthood with any health at all because I gave my body so little to work with during those adolescent years.

Nutrition clearly wasn't on my mind back then but what I did think about—constantly—was how urgently I wanted to eat all the time and how miserable I was about my body. I went on with my education, my career, and my life in general, but eating thoroughly dominated my inner world until the age of 43. I can't recall any moment of peace and sanity with food ever before that time. It was a constant battle of obsessing about eating, eating bizarre types and quantities of food, and being wracked by shame and embarrassment. It seemed it was simply my fate always to be enslaved by relentless urges to eat destructively, despite how desperately I wanted it to be different. Few would have guessed at my torment in my adult years because I always managed to stay at a healthy *looking* weight, though I constantly bounced around within a 15-pound range.

Thanks to the work of Dr. Gregory Boothroyd,[1] that all changed in 2001. After learning his therapeutic technique for the elimination of self-defeating behaviors, I decided to try it on my compulsive overeating.

I expected nothing, of course. *Sure*, I thought. *Let's do this on eating. R-i-g-h-t.* I was amazed, therefore, when it caused something inside me to shift, helping me to see food differently than I ever had before. I recall no turning point in my life before or since that could match the feeling I had when I realized I could actually be free from the torment after all.

In the years since I've enjoyed greater clarity and peace with food, I have studied the topic of overeating from various angles: how it works, what encourages or supports it from within and without, its various impacts, and the science of the brain behind it all. I have shared this growing body of information on the topic with individual clients and in community education seminars along the way. When I updated and reorganized the material in 2015, I realized that it had grown beyond the scope of a time-limited seminar, and that it had evolved into a unique enough approach to the problem to warrant greater public exposure. For those reasons, this book came into being.

I hope to show you why it's no mystery that most of us now struggle with overeating. When you understand why it has happened, you are in a far stronger position to change your life for the better, for good. What that means is that you'll feel more in control of what you do and why you do it, and therefore better able to live the life you want the most, whatever that is.

The material in this book is arranged to give you the context that will help the central ideas to make the most sense as you get to them. For that reason, I recommend going through the book from beginning to end rather than sampling randomly; you may miss some important connections if you take the information out of sequence.

My greatest hope is that this work brings you closer to finding your own freedom with food. It takes some adjusting to create and maintain a life with food that is healthy *and* happy, but it can be done. It is one of the most important victories you can achieve in this life.

Wishing you peace,
Elizabeth Babcock, LCSW
July 2016

Part One

Unintended Consequences of Modern Life

Chapter 1
The Deep Desire to Be Normal

I just want to be able to eat like a normal person!
I know what to do but I just don't do it.
What's wrong with me??

If you are like most overeaters, this is how you talk to yourself a lot of the time. You may also suspect that you are unusually pathological in this regard, that there is some shred of hope for others who overeat, but not for you. You will soon learn not only that there is hope for you, but that your difficulties with food are due to the fact that you are *completely* normal.

What is abnormal, historically speaking, is the way we now live. In the course of just a few decades, we have adopted lifestyle changes that seemed like good ideas at the time, but which actually created an unprecedented, population-wide wave of destructive food behaviors.

Roughly 69% of US adults are overweight and half of those are obese as of 2012,[1] the most recent year for which information was available at the time of this writing. Many others struggle to control themselves with food but since they manage to maintain a healthy weight, they don't show up in any statistics. Still more fall into the dangerous addictions of anorexia and bulimia. The fact is that people with no food problems of any kind are now the exception, and decidedly so.

If the vast majority of the population now has food problems, there is something in play that affects most people in a similar way. *You* have the food issues that you have because this is what happens to normal human beings in certain, highly specific conditions. Those conditions— low physical activity and constant access to hyperpalatable food— happen to be the cornerstones of the lifestyle so diligently pursued by most nations in the developed (and developing) world.

When you understand what it is about the way we live that affects most normal people the way it does, the solutions become clear. The

3

way out is simple though not easy, because it is hard to adopt new patterns when most people around you are clinging to the old ones and encouraging you to join them. This is especially true if some of those people are those you love the most, as is often the case.

So, what have we been doing in recent decades that has so many of us working against our own best interests, despite knowing and wanting better for ourselves?

Chapter 2
So Much Eating

While food has an ever growing range of roles in our lives, the boundaries around its general use are dwindling away. These two trends are significant in the problems many of us now have with overeating, and they have been developing in various areas of our lives at the same time. They have been changing at such a rapid rate that most of our population has been unable to adapt and keep up, as evidenced by the epidemic of disordered eating.

Eating as Our Primary Social Activity
Including food in our social plans is not only enjoyable but may meet a practical need. If you spend an extended amount of time together, somebody's likely to get hungry at some point, so you'll have to plan for what, when, and how you're going to eat. So far, so good.

The problem is that over time, many of us have shifted from having food as *part* of our shared activities to making food the *focus* of them.

Many of my clients, for example, can recall when they used to get together with friends to do something fun, often eating in conjunction with their primary plans. Now they just get together to eat.[1] Instead of sharing an activity and then grabbing some lunch, they just meet for lunch. Instead of going for an afternoon walk, they spend the afternoon chatting at a coffee house. They are not only missing out on the movement and experience of the activities they used to share, but are also sitting more and eating more—a lot more.

It barely seems possible now for two or more people to consider spending any amount of time together for any reason without including provisions for eating while they're at it.

It is considered negligent to host or plan any activity involving others that does not include food of some kind, no matter how brief the activity is or how little it has to do with eating. Food has always been an

5

integral part of how we interact and bond, but the social pressure around this aspect of its use seems to have increased dramatically in recent times.

Special Occasions All the Time

Food has always been an important part of how we bond as families and as societies. Special meals have long been a predictable marker of entertaining as well as the celebration of various life milestones and special occasions throughout the year.

The problem is that there are now so *many* events that we see as special occasions befitting an abundance of food and a reason to "take a day off" from whatever food-management efforts we may be making.

We start with New Year's, then on to the Super Bowl, followed shortly by Valentine's Day, St. Patrick's Day, and then Easter. There's a short stretch to the Memorial Day picnic, then the graduation parties that will bridge the gap to the Fourth of July. We have a pause before Labor Day festivities, then a bit of a breather before Halloween.

From there, it's full blast into the six straight weeks of winter parties and holidays that will bring us once again to the New Year, which we may greet with a couple more pounds than last time. And that's without taking into account the various game-day parties, birthdays, weddings, anniversaries and such that are sprinkled throughout the year.

We treat each of these occasions as a rare, special event when cumulatively, they can easily happen a couple of times monthly or more, all year long. You might manage damage-free enjoyment of a *few* food free-for-alls in a year, but not one every few weeks. Beware the tendency to invoke "special occasion rules" for events that, as a general class, actually happen quite often.

Eating for Any Reason or No Reason at All

The most basic purpose of food is to provide fuel and nutrition for the body, but overeaters most often use it for emotional self-regulation and personal entertainment. This starts in toddlerhood as children become responsive to social cues and positive reinforcement, and develop the natural tendency to copy behavior they see in others.[2]

Parents quickly learn that the easiest way to comfort, distract, entertain or reward a child is with food, and most will assure that they always have snacks on hand for these needs. The unintentional lesson to the child is that food is the all-purpose, go-to strategy for anything and everything. Those who internalize this lesson at an impressionable age risk spending the remainder of their lives trying to manage a deep-seated urge to go to food for every discomfort or imbalance.

Habitual use of food for emotional needs removes a boundary that would otherwise naturally keep the eating in check. If you're eating primarily for physical needs, the body needs just so much and that's the end of it until the next time that hunger develops.

By comparison, emotional needs are potentially endless; there is no clear stopping point when you eat that way other than becoming physically uncomfortable or simply running out of food. Worse, food does not even help with these needs other than in an illusory, all-too-brief way. No amount of food will heal emotional pain, but vast quantities of it get consumed in the futile attempt to do just that.

More is Better, Right?
Everything about our food, it seems, has been expanding since the 1970s. In addition to bigger portions, we also have an increasing variety of novel food products from which to choose, most of which have much greater caloric density per bite than the foods of the past.

We snack and graze throughout most of each day on these new products in addition to using them to augment or replace our meals. The caloric density combines with frequency of intake to create a simple but serious mathematical problem: our caloric intake has skyrocketed compared to that of past generations.

We have more options for obtaining food than ever before. We have larger and more diversified supermarkets, intentionally laid out in ways that encourage impulse buying. Hundreds of thousands of restaurants compete for market share, spending huge advertising budgets on commercials that—again—are meant to trigger us into impulse buying. Many of these restaurants have helpfully installed drive-throughs and instituted curbside pick-up programs, making it as easy as possible for us to obtain their high-calorie food.

The challenge of all this is twofold. First, all these new and bigger options mean that food literally looms larger in our psychological worlds. It is hard *not* to think about eating constantly when food has such an overwhelming physical presence in our lives. More specifically though, we naturally respond to an abundance of food with more eating.[3,4] We are triggered by larger quantities and by greater variety,[5] and are exposed to more of both now than has previously been experienced by any population group in human history.

Because we are the first to experience this kind of abundance, we are learning the hard way that normal human beings don't cope well in these conditions.

The Loss of Food-Free Space in Our Lives

Talk to people from your parents' or grandparents' generations and you'll quickly learn that most meals used to be consumed at home, only in kitchens and dining rooms, and most often at designated mealtimes. There was occasional snacking but mostly, people were otherwise occupied the rest of the time, seldom combining eating with other activities.

Compare this to the homes of today where it is normal not only to eat in any room of the house at any time, but while doing many other things like watching TV, working online, and taking care of various household tasks. And that's if food is even eaten at home at all.

Americans in 2012 were spending 43% of their food budget on food from outside the home,[6] which represents many meals each week eaten out, carried in, or eaten in the car. This lack of structure around eating was unheard of in your grandparents' time but, as with all the other changes noted earlier in this chapter, if you were born any time after about 1970, it is all you have ever known.

Workplaces have undergone a similar transformation. Food at work was once generally restricted to planned lunchtimes or breaks, most often in an employee cafeteria, break room, or lounge. Recent decades have seen the normalization of eating meals at one's desk or other work station, which has morphed further into grazing on snacks throughout the day.

The workplace, then, is another space in which food used to show up only in structured, predictable ways, but where it has now become fully integrated into most that we do there. Actually, the workplace has become a place of rather intense food *pressure* for many people, as someone always seems to be bringing in goodies, there's often a birthday or other special occasion to celebrate, and even meetings often involve munchies of some kind.

Why should you think about changes like these? Because there was no major obesity problem in America when more structured practices were in place, and that is not a coincidence.

For most of human history, there have been natural limits around food. You were lucky to find enough, and that was the limit. You couldn't have an overeating problem if there wasn't a reliable excess of food available.

As we got better at stabilizing the food supply, we lived for generations with social conventions that maintained artificial limits around food. There were times and places for it as described above, and no expectation or habit of large portions. While it was becoming easier to develop overeating patterns as food supplies became more reliable, relatively few people did because social norms did not support it.

In a single human lifetime—which happens to coincide with yours—we have done away with nearly every social convention that used to put boundaries around reliably available food. Instead, we now actually *promote* the use of food with few limits at all.

Whatever else you may say about times past, having more limits around food helped us all to stay more easily in check. Removing them has left us with the relatively new need for consistent, purposeful self-management with food. You will see later why most of us are failing so miserably at this (and also how to approach it much more effectively).

It is vital to understand just how inexperienced humanity is with our current practices when you are trying to figure out where food really belongs in your life. These practices may be all you have ever known—or at least all you've done now for many years—but they are vanishingly new in the long timeline of human existence.

The point is that the way we are with food today bears no resemblance to how human beings have been with food ever before. You may believe that your familiar food practices are "normal," but the reality is that we are in uncharted territory.[7] Remember that, and it may be easier to see what you need to do to get the food part of your life to start making a lot more sense.

Chapter 3
So Little Food

Something fascinating has been happening to our food supply—there seems to be a lot less actual food in it than there used to be. Look at the ingredient list on any can, box, bag, bottle or carton that you have in your kitchen and you will most likely see some ingredients that you don't really understand. You also won't be able to find or purchase them in your local grocery store. The fact that it's hard to guess the true nature of such ingredients is a bad sign, because real food is not confusing.

All real food was at one time a living thing—plant or animal—most likely with a name you recognize; all else is essentially a science project. If you have any doubt, do some Internet searches on ingredient list terms that you don't understand, and see what you think of what you find. Are these substances that you would ever have a reason to seek out for yourself? Do you know enough about them to have an informed opinion? Do you find yourself kind of not wanting to know?

It is common sense to keep things that aren't food out of your body, because it could be dangerous to have them there. It would seldom occur to you to eat soap or paper towels or hand lotion, for example, and nobody (absent certain mental health issues) would want to anyway because those items aren't enjoyable to eat.

But what if those same products tasted great and had a texture you found irresistible?

Eating Products Instead of Food

Over the past century, what we eat has increasingly come from factories rather than farms. Manufacturers take a variety of ingredients, some of which are food and some of which are not, and combine them into the products they sell. They do this with awareness that we seek products that are tasty, cheap, portable, convenient, and which will store well.

Some amount of manufactured food helps a lot in keeping a stable food supply for a very large population. To meet our need for enough affordable, tasty, portable, convenient food for everyone,[1] we probably have to tolerate some level of additives in the supply.

It's a fine line because for the most part, the more manufactured (altered) a food product is, the less it is composed of elements that are recognizable and beneficial to our bodies. Most industrial processing— while it is creating the cheap, tasty, convenient food that we want—is reducing the nutritional value of that food along the way.

There is more in play, however, than just compromising on quality a bit in order to ensure adequate quantity. Manufacturers seek to maximize profits, which they accomplish by reducing the cost of production and by increasing sales.

Reducing costs means looking for economies of scale, but it also means using cheaper ingredients. You get a cheaper and longer lasting product if it is fruit *flavored*, for example, than if it is created from actual fruit.

How do you get the flavor without the food it comes from? Additives.[2] So we started with food that we compromised a bit in order to be able to make enough of it, and now we've compromised it a little more to save money on flavoring. It's slightly less food-like than it was before.

What's better than figuring out how to use cheaper substances to copy what we like in the wild? Figuring out how to use those substances to create things we like even *more*. On the face of it, cheaper and better seems like a great outcome. We've created amped-up versions of the natural flavors we crave and have also invented entirely new ones; we've developed whole new classes of food textures that are far more entertaining than anything you'd find out in the wild.

Each time we make the flavor more delicious or the texture more compelling, our product contains less food and more additives. At the extreme, we have some products that are barely food at all; the snack category is particularly well known for this.

Thanks to additives, a lot of our food is now much cheaper yet also has an impressive "wow factor." It's hardly food anymore but it's irresistible,[3] so it flies off the shelves anyway. Voilà! There are the increased sales the manufacturers were hoping for.

We may love the stuff, but there's little else to say for it. It's addictive, bizarrely high in calories and at best, nutritionally marginal. It's full of substances without enough of a track record for us to know what their long-term impact will be. The necessary research is

11

underway right now, by the way; you and your family are voluntary subjects. You never gave your informed consent to participate in this research, but you agree to it every time you buy one of these products.

The availability of so many food-like products has made food selection seem more complicated, but there have been various attempts to help us sort through the fantastic array of choices we have.

One example is the Guiding Stars program implemented by the Hannaford Brothers Supermarkets (New England) in 2006.[4] The program is simple enough, sorting food for consumers as follows: a one-star rating means the nutritional content is "good," two stars is "better," and three stars is "best." It is noteworthy that when this program was applied to the 25,500 products then available in that supermarket chain, a full 72% of the items rated no stars at all.[5] That was nine years ago at the time of this writing, and the profusion of confusing, addictive, edible products has only grown since then.

This is important because these are the products that, in addition to compromising our health, cause us to lose control of our eating. We have become a population of people who are simultaneously overfed and malnourished, cruelly suffering the health consequences of both.

Outsourcing Our Food

The consumption of more and more manufactured foods is part of a larger issue, that of steadily turning over more responsibility for our families' food to profit-seeking entities outside the home.

The average American in the 1950s most often ate home-prepared whole foods because that was what was readily available. Processed foods were just entering the mainstream market and were viewed by many with disdain, as low-grade substitutes for the real thing. Eating out was rare.

From that point to the present, processed products have become the primary staple foods in most American homes,[6] and eating out regularly has become quite common. Search nutritional information on any restaurant you plan to visit and you will be shocked by the caloric density and sodium content of most of your options.

This means that no matter where most of us are eating now, we are choosing products in which corners have been cut to shave costs, while additives have been used to boost the flavor off the charts so that we'll always want to come back for more.

The nutritional and economic impacts of these trends are concrete enough, but there is another consequence which, though harder to quantify, is at least as important. We are losing our innate understanding of what food is, where it comes from, how to evaluate it, how to select and prepare it, and how it fits into our lives.

We are losing the herd knowledge accumulated by countless generations over the past 40,000 years (or more),[7] and are thus becoming incompetent at the basic natural task of feeding ourselves.[8] At the risk of stating the obvious, this is an astounding development.

How can we hope to manage our eating if we lose our basic understanding of food?

Chapter 4
Still Life

No book on overeating is complete without including a look at the place of physical activity in our lives. If you have the dieting mindset shared by most Americans, you might assume this is about working off more calories or about more effective health management in general. Those effects do matter, of course, but there is a more fundamental reason why overeaters in particular need to think hard about this:

If you are not moderately active on a fairly consistent basis, it is nearly impossible to keep your head screwed on straight about eating.

There is a powerful connection between regular exercise and the ability to maintain focus with food. It's hard to maintain one without the other; if you lose track of one, the other tends to fall away soon after. Deep down, you probably already know this. For that reason, I urge you to read on and consider the information that follows.

The Loss of Movement in Modern Life
It is only recently in American history that most of us have had the ability to choose a sedentary way of life. From 1910 to 2000, the majority of our workforce shifted from brute force work like farming, mining, and manufacturing to professional, technical, clerical, and sales jobs.[1]

It was a sign of progress and improving quality of life that we were able to create work that was easier and safer than much of what had come before, but it did result in the removal of much physical activity from our lives.

We have mirrored this shift in our leisure time as well. Many of us have left behind the more physically oriented hobbies of the past in favor of many hours now spent online. It's hard to know whether we're losing interest in being more physically involved in our lives or whether

14

it is simply a matter of competing interests which are incompatible with being up and moving around.

In any event, most of us now spend our lives sitting, often punctuated only by brief strolls to get to another room or to get to and from our cars. We move some for basic household tasks and errands and that may *feel* like being busy, but that doesn't usually translate into much actual physical activity; the fact is that we move dramatically less than has any previous generation. It took a great deal of innovation to create a way of life in which it is actually possible to move too little, but as soon as we had that choice, we seized it.

Physical activity has become such an oddity in our lives that we have a special name for it now—"exercise"—and we do it mostly in specially designed places—fitness centers, health clubs and gyms—rather than experiencing it as the natural part of daily life that it always was until the late 20th century. We now have to make a point to think about it, plan for it, and schedule around it, which would have been inconceivable to people from just a couple of generations ago.

Every physical system we have, it seems, operates more effectively when regularly used.[2,3] Your body shows you this when you feel better as a result of having moved around even a little more than usual if you are normally sedentary.

It is very easy in our fast-paced world, however, to overlook how little we move on most days. It is also easy to feel that there is just no time to fit it in anywhere. The price that we pay for this creeps up on us incrementally, causing our quality of life to dwindle without us even noticing it until the losses have become quite pronounced.

The High Price of Low Activity Levels
The most obvious cost of moving too little is that far fewer calories get burned. This is particularly damaging when combined—as it usually is—with the overconsumption of high-calorie foods. The outcome of that particular math is terrible, but is barely the beginning of the price we pay for being too still.

Our bodies operate on the use-it-or-lose-it principle.[4] The less we move, the harder it becomes *to* move, for a variety of reasons. Range and ease of motion are compromised as muscles and tendons get tighter and shorter from lack of use. Aerobic condition falls, reducing endurance. Muscles lose condition, reducing both strength and endurance. Coordination and balance degrade due to simple lack of practice, in addition to the normal losses to those systems which occur with aging.[5] Immune system function is compromised as the body falls further and further out of condition,[6] thus being less able to protect, repair and maintain itself (By the way, isn't it amazing that our bodies can actually *fix* themselves?!).

You start spending more of your time coping with opportunistic infections, more time getting over them, and more time just feeling "off." Pain levels tend to increase on more sedentary days; this dampens interest in moving, fueling the vicious cycle of escalating and longer-lasting pain.

Options for managing and enjoying life are severely reduced if you are less able to move. There are fewer ways to make life interesting, challenging, and fun. There are fewer ways to share memorable bonding experiences with friends and loved ones. There are fewer ways to blow off steam when you're stressed. There is simply much less of most things that make life worthwhile.

Being sedentary into your 50s and beyond will steal your ability to walk without assistive devices many years sooner than necessary. It can become the factor that determines whether or not you remain independent as you age.

Brain health suffers far more than most people might realize. Physical activity is now recognized as one of the most powerful tools you have for maintaining your brain as you age. Inadequate levels of activity are associated with incremental deterioration of memory, mood, and general mental sharpness; sedentary people are at greater risk for dementia, and for getting it earlier.[7]

In short, moving too little means a less enjoyable and more stressful life today, and sets the stage for senior years that are unnecessarily limited, painful, and frustrating. This means that you live with a higher baseline stress level at all times which, whether or not you are aware of it, creates a nagging need for emotional relief. That leads, of course, to frequent urges to eat for comfort.

And *that* is why you need to keep moving if you want any hope of controlling your drive to overeat.

A Dangerous New Syndrome

There is a specific element of moving too little which deserves special mention, and that is the issue of sitting too much. Lack of exercise increases the risk of cardiovascular disease, type 2 diabetes, and various cancers, but if you regularly sit for many uninterrupted hours at a time, that risk is increased even further.[8]

Unfortunately, you can*not* compensate for this additional risk with regular exercise if you spend most of the rest of your time sitting,[9] and those who try have even been referred to as "active couch potatoes."[10] Every year, millions of people die prematurely due to chronic diseases that were triggered or exacerbated by an overly sedentary way of life. We lose so many people this way that Sedentary Death Syndrome[11] is the term often used to describe the cause of such deaths.

Whether or not you ever adopt a consistent pattern of actual exercise, the hazards of sitting too much can be avoided simply by incorporating more general movement into the rest of your day. Get up often, stand when you can, walk when you can, stretch when you can, and create opportunities for these simple acts all day long. Seldom in life will you encounter a problem so serious that is so easy to solve.

Scientific research and new buzzwords aside, we probably all have life experience that shows us we feel better when we are more active than we do when we are more sedentary. In the end, that is all the information you really need.

Chapter 5
Living Longer, Aging Faster

Longevity statistics might not feel like the most fascinating topic in the world, but they provide an important perspective at this point in our story. Lifespan here in the US, for example, has increased steadily throughout our history.[1]

We've gotten this far by stabilizing the availability of food and clean water, improving general sanitation, vaccinating against infectious disease, smoking less, and developing a variety of medical advances that have extended and improved quality of life.[2] Today's longevity is a product of changes and innovations from the past, slowly rippling their way forward through time.

What we do today then, will ripple forward through time to create the longevity experienced by our descendants. It can be tempting to think that we will always live longer and things will always get better no matter what simply because in our lifetimes, that's been true.

The recent spike in obesity rates,[3] however, is now reversing many of the health gains we previously worked so hard to achieve. It is obesity and its medical consequences that threaten the lifespan of today's children,[4] along with degrading the general health in most other age groups compared to just 15 years ago.[5] We are now in the novel position of witnessing the first large-scale reversal of public health in our history.

Our population has begun to experience accelerated aging even as our longevity—for now—continues to rise. We see increasing incidence of disability in younger and younger adults,[6] which means that while we're gaining years of life, we're simultaneously losing *healthy* years. The costs in terms of reduced quality of life and increasing medical expense promise to be staggering for most of us now in adulthood, but what about our kids?

We see children developing diseases previously known only in adults: conditions like cardiovascular disease, type 2 diabetes, bone and joint problems, sleep apnea, fatty liver disease, and depression.[7,8]

We are in uncharted territory as pediatricians scramble to become more conversant in medical issues they weren't supposed to see, and we begin to find out the hard way what it means for human beings to be treated for these conditions beginning in childhood rather than in middle or older age.

How does it affect us to take the necessary medications for these conditions decades longer than was ever intended or studied? What happens when we use adult medications on children during crucial times in their development?

We don't know, but we are forced to try it and see how it plays out over time. However grim the eventual disability risk for today's adults, it is considerably worse for today's children. It can't turn out well when you're saddled with coronary artery disease or type 2 diabetes before you've finished high school, for example, and we now have lots of kids on exactly that trajectory.

This is clearly not a position we want to be in. Nobody meant for it to turn out this way, yet here we are.

While our current way of life sets the stage for this mess, few of us (with the noteworthy exception of children) are forced to choose it. Most of us have access to better food than we usually eat and more activity than we usually pursue. Most of us have the personal experience to know that we feel better when we make higher quality choices for ourselves, yet we don't make them with much consistency.

On the surface, this makes no sense at all. That just means that the surface is not the right place to search for an explanation.

Chapter 6
The Obvious Question

It's a curious thing when a huge population adopts a disease-promoting way of life, sees the danger, agonizes over it at length, then continues to do it anyway. If you look to our origins, the explanation becomes clear.

Why We Keep Eating Destructively
The reality for most of humanity—as for most animal life on Earth—has always been the struggle to find enough food to survive. We were here long before there were cities and suburbs, factory farms and supermarkets. In an undeveloped environment, food insecurity is the norm and you had better exploit every opportunity for eating that you get since you never know what's coming next, if anything.

The drive to eat whatever you can, whenever you can, makes perfect sense when there's not enough food available. Bring that same drive into a setting where high-calorie food is constantly available, and you can begin to see the problem.

Our dilemma is intensified by the fact that so much of our food supply is now organized around the flavors of sugar, salt, and fat, present in processed foods at concentrations much higher than anything that can be found in nature. This has not occurred by accident, of course. Those flavors are the foundation of our processed foods simply because we like them so much. As a successful species taking control of its food supply, it is predictable that we would skew our food toward the flavors that we prefer.

It's likely that we have those particular preferences because, in conditions of food insecurity, they promote survival. The desire for sugar and fat lead us to the higher-calorie food sources that are critical when you need to make sure you are getting enough to support life. The taste for sugar also leads us toward the essential nutrients found in fruits. Sodium is generally available at low levels in whole foods, fitting nicely with the fact that trace quantities of it are essential to life.[1] If we tend toward saltier-tasting foods in the wild, it guarantees that we'll get the minimal amount of sodium that we need.

The problem is that our abundant supply of manufactured food confronts us with sugar, salt and fat in quantities and intensities that bear no resemblance to anything we could find in an undeveloped environment. We are biologically unprepared for dealing with this level of availability, so most of us will predictably lose control of our eating when consuming foods based on these flavors.[2]

We've done it to ourselves, unfortunately. It is a primary drive to secure as much food as possible, so we naturally engineered our lives to create maximum food security. With food now readily available to most of us at all times, we have to manage the drive for food acquisition very intentionally; we have to choose to stop eating even though there is still food available.

This choice is new, and doesn't come naturally to most of us because it's a skill we might never need in the wild. It's a recent requirement of modern life, and based on the overwhelming prevalence of eating and weight problems in our country, most of us have not adapted to this new challenge. If you feel like you are eating without brakes, that may not be far from the truth.

Why We Avoid Exercise When We Know Better
Life in the wild can be something of a grind. Every basic need we have—food, water, shelter, safety—requires work. Sometimes it's a lot of work, and it's required almost every day.

You need to conserve energy as much as possible to assure that you have it when necessary for acquiring food, fending off or evading predators, and keeping up with the basic maintenance tasks of life. You don't have to be motivated to move in such circumstances because you have no choice but to move quite a lot—if you don't, you die. *There's* your motivation.

Obviously then, another goal we had in creating a more comfortable life was to reduce the level of brute force effort it requires. We've therefore been busily engineering away the dangerous, tedious, exhausting work of our lives. After millennia of having to keep working no matter how tired you get, it's nice to be able to rest when you want to.

As it turns out, however, we've been too successful for our own good. We are physiologically adapted to survival in the untamed world we so recently left behind. Our bodies are optimized for regular movement and work, as evidenced by the fact that they require it for good health. Take away too much of the physicality of life, and health slowly begins to decline.

Here again in modern life, we have unwittingly created the need for a choice we are not wired to make: to move on purpose for its own sake, rather than because we have to. After millennia of seeking rest opportunities whenever possible and having that work quite well for our survival as a species, we now find ourselves having to choose the opposite. Small wonder most of us are so resistant to the idea.

The Critical Inversion

The elements above combine in a disastrous way. Consider two aspects of our lives:

- One occurs only in certain places and at certain times, with the expectation of specific limits.

- The other occurs almost anywhere, almost any time.

The first used to describe how we eat and the second used to describe our physical activity, but that has changed. It used to be movement that was fully integrated into most of our waking hours, but now it's eating.

For most of humanity across the ages, life has involved a little eating and a lot of activity; there was simply no other choice. In less than one human lifetime, we've inverted the ratio. We've done this because, having the capacity to manipulate our world, we prioritized and innovated based on our instinctual drives. Well, of course we did. What else would we ever do?

Unfortunately for us, we've been able to transcend some boundaries we actually needed. The act of building around our drives drastically reduced the natural limitations (scarce food, life requiring a lot of work) that once kept those drives in check. The results speak for themselves.

Part Two

The Deep Origins of Overeating
and
Why Willpower Can't Save the Day

Chapter 7
It's All About Your Brain

Lest you fear this book is about to veer into boring, incomprehensible scientific jargon, rest assured that it is not. You just need to know a bit about three general areas of the brain, how those areas function,[1] and the implications of that information for food management in modern life. Once you understand how this all fits together, everything else you need to know and do will make sense.

The Brainstem

Brains are built from the bottom up, with the brainstem being the oldest, most essential part of the brain. The brainstem we have now is quite similar to those currently in use by all of today's backboned creatures.[2] Like theirs, ours sits at the top of the spinal cord, regulating life support functions like the beating of the heart, breathing, digestion, and maintenance of blood pressure.

The brainstem is not a source of learning or personality; it just keeps the basics going. You see it in operation in simpler vertebrates like fish, which have only the brainstem and a few additional brain structures for sensing and reacting to environmental stimuli. Creatures at this level are complex organisms, but their behavior is primarily reflexive and instinctual in nature; they show little individuality. One goldfish, for example, is behaviorally about the same as any other.

The Limbic System

As life forms become more complex, the brain continues to develop beyond the brainstem. The next layer of structures is the limbic system,[3] often referred to as the emotional brain or emotional system.

In order to succeed as a species, we need to be motivated to behave in ways that will help us and to avoid behaviors that will hurt us; we also need to figure out which is which. The emotional brain generates the feelings that make this analysis possible, evaluating elements of the environment and generally categorizing them as beneficial, problematic, or unimportant.

These assessments are performed almost instantly as needed, as befits decisions related to survival. They are based on the perception of the challenge or opportunity in question, the results that seem most readily associated with it, and the emotions triggered by those results. This information then gets stored into memory where it becomes the basis of future behavior.[4]

The emotional system is the first level of the brain where learning begins to occur, but it is a very rudimentary, associations-based kind of learning: *I like this—it's a good thing that I want more of. I don't like that—it's a bad thing that I want to avoid.*

Once the emotional system has categorized something one way or the other, it tends to stick with that initial impression for quick future reference rather than repeatedly re-evaluating at each additional encounter. Once you've identified a preferred food, for example, you will automatically seek it out when possible rather than continuing to decide each time whether you still like it or not.

Animals with this level of brain functioning show general similarity within their species while displaying individual differences. For example, certain behaviors are essentially universal among housecats, yet each one has a clearly distinct personality.

The same can be said of any of the mammals with whom we tend to share our lives. It can, for that matter, be said of us even though this is not where our brain development plateaus.

The emotional brain is necessarily quite powerful, as its primary function is to help us navigate and survive in an unforgiving and unpredictable environment. In humans, though, it does much more than simply enhance survival; it is where your experience of life registers because it is where you *feel*, and is the origin of much that is uniquely you.

When you experience satisfaction, joy, love, pain, boredom, purpose, anger, despair, wonder, or any of the other feelings that are part of being human, the emotional brain is where they are all felt.

Remember that for later.

The Cerebral Cortex

The cerebral cortex is the newest and outermost part of the brain, often referred to simply as the cortex or more colloquially, the thinking brain. It is that layer of gray matter with many folds which is so prominent in whole-brain photos and illustrations, and is the tissue which supports the most sophisticated functioning in the brain.

Unlike the emotional system which focuses only on this moment, the cortex takes in this moment as part of a much longer timeline. The emotional brain reacts to what *is*, while the cortex imagines and creates what *could be*.

The cortex can conceive and follow through on plans that may take months or even years to complete, because it is able to imagine the benefits to come despite possibly lower rewards in the present.[5]

The cortex learns from experience, but it also learns by studying its environment and evaluating how to optimize it. Its powers of reasoning, deduction, imagination and innovation allow us to develop solutions to complex problems. The cortex empowers us to change the present and the future, altering the course of our own lives.[6]

Despite these remarkable capabilities, the cortex can be overridden by the lower parts of the brain that, while less sophisticated, are more immediately necessary to survival in the wild. The irony of the cortex is that it has both the broadest capabilities and the least power in the system.[7]

Implications

Life turns out the best when the various areas of the brain work together in a coordinated fashion that maximizes the strengths of each. The rules of the natural world generally promote the seamless operation of the brain as a whole, but that isn't the world where we now live.

A complication of our current lifestyle is that, for reasons that make no sense in the wild, the rules for survival have drastically changed. This isn't a problem for the brainstem, which is more about internal maintenance than about what's going on outside the body. It's also not a problem for the cortex, which is capable of reorienting and altering strategy at any time based on changing needs and information.

Where the new rules of survival go horribly wrong is in the emotional brain. The emotional brain is how we experience all the very best parts of life—it is important to always remember and be grateful for that. However, it is also a reactive, short-sighted, somewhat stubborn system with tendencies that work well most of the time in the wild, but which fail most of the time in the world we have worked so hard to create for ourselves.

As much as we love our comforts, pleasures and conveniences, they create a setting in which the functioning of our emotional brain now works at cross purposes to our survival rather than enhancing it. We experience this when we feel powerless in the face of an urge to overeat or do anything else that we know will ultimately be harmful. We may know deeply that a choice we're considering is going to end badly, yet feel unable to stop ourselves. We feel weak, undisciplined, despicable, and maybe even somewhat insane—*who in their right mind would do this?*—yet we can't stop.

There is actually a perfectly good explanation for this. To see how it works, we must have a deeper understanding of the realities and vulnerabilities of this powerful part of the brain.

Chapter 8
The Emotional Brain Revealed

Look no further than the nearest dog or cat to see most of what you need to know about the emotional brain. Like us, our pets have well-developed and powerful limbic systems but while our brains go on to develop much further, theirs do so only minimally. As a result, their behaviors and patterns nicely demonstrate how an emotional-brain-based life is lived.

We might like to think that our pets live on our terms, but the reality is that we have to work around them and have simply chosen the animals that require the least adjustment on our part. Dogs and cats are the most popular pets not just because they (usually) have such pleasing personalities, but because their natural behavioral tendencies are the easiest ones for us to live with. They are the most likely to be safe, enjoyable live-in companions for our families, eliminating their waste where we hope they will, and perhaps leaving most of our belongings unmolested.

The reason any number of other available animals have never caught on as pets is that we just can't adjust to the ways they tend to behave. If you doubt this, spend some time attempting to live with, say, a groundhog.

The point is that as much as we love them and as smart as we often think they are, our pets have only a limited, drive-based repertoire of responses. Their emotional brains are what give them the personalities we cherish, along with the following general characteristics:

- If they really want to do something, you can't dissuade them unless you make the act immediately unpleasant for them or offer them an equally appealing alternative. Otherwise, you have to distract them until they forget about it, make it impossible for them to follow through, or just put up with them doing whatever it is.

- If they don't want to do something, you can't change that, either. You have to find a way to trick or force them into doing it, or just give up and live without it happening at all.

- They react strongly and without deliberation to perceived opportunities and threats, based only on what motivates them the most right in the moment (unless they've received considerable training for alternative behaviors). Their concept of the future is limited at best, so they have little capacity for planning and strategy. Their thinking would sound like, *I want this!* or, *I need to get away!* rather than, *I can see how this is going to turn out and will choose accordingly.*

- They can only make connections between actions and results that occur nearly simultaneously. Most cause and effect relationships are beyond their comprehension because they have so little ability to understand how this moment relates to any other moment in time, be it five minutes ago or five minutes from now.

Now, consider the characteristics above as you think about the part of you that urgently goes after food in ways that repeatedly sabotage your health and peace of mind:

- If you really want to eat something, you can't stop wanting it unless it is somehow made immediately unpleasant (like the snack you're obsessing over until you're able to squirt dishwashing liquid all over it) or you can identify an equally appealing alternative. Otherwise, you have to distract yourself and hope you can forget about it, make it impossible to obtain, or just give up and eat it so that at least the inner torment will stop.

- If you don't want to do something (like exercising regularly), you can't make yourself want it even though you believe you should. You have to find a way to trick, bargain, or force yourself into it, or just give it up so that at least you're not fighting with yourself over it anymore.

- You are triggered rapidly and intensely by your most tempting foods. You quickly lose your will to resist them or to have them in moderation. You'd like to be more deliberative in those moments—you truly would—but you just can't do it.

- Your strongest feelings are based on how much you do or don't want to do something *right now*. Part of you knows you'll feel bad about this later, but that fails to outweigh the urgency you feel in the moment. You wonder how you could possibly not have learned the lesson yet after all the times it has gone this way before.

There you go—you've just met your emotional brain. As frustrated as you may presently feel with it, remember that this system works extremely well in settings of scarcity and hardship, which is all most of humanity has ever known until quite recently. It has a lot to do with our surviving and thriving enough to be here now.

In fact, we as a species have been so spectacularly successful that we've been able to remake our world, a world in which—ironically—the emotional brain is now tragically out of its element. In order to appreciate why that is so, it pays to understand some fundamentals about how this part of you works.

Chapter 9
Six Important Things to Know
About Your Emotional Brain

It is a Powerful Rapid-Response System
The emotional brain is first in line after the brainstem to receive most incoming sensory information. Since it's adapted to dealing with spontaneous life-or-death challenges in an unforgiving environment, its reaction speed is far greater than that of the cortex.

Because it is more essential to immediate survival, it has the power to override the cortex altogether if it is triggered enough. In situations where pausing to think could be what gets you killed, this is a good thing. A practical consideration here is that the emotional brain can begin to react to incoming information and lock out the cortex before the cortex even has a chance to get in the game.

Being confronted with highly appealing food is not a life-or-death event, but it can cause intense reactivity in the emotional system just the same. Anything that triggers the emotional brain—the sight, smell, mention, or mere thought of certain foods—can activate the mechanisms that begin to lock out the cortex.

For successful food management in the modern world, you must minimize those circumstances in which your emotional brain can start to spin up and take over before your cortex can save the day.

It Prioritizes the Present
Life in the wild is all about surviving the moment and helping one's offspring to do the same, so the emotional brain is anchored in the present. It does not readily learn from delayed consequences nor does it readily embrace delayed gratification; these inputs are too far removed in time to motivate it to a meaningful degree.

It reacts the most to whatever is most immediate, which is why you're drawn so powerfully to a trigger food rather than to the less tangible results of the more distant future. The tortured debate in your head might sound like, *This is going to be so great—I can't wait!*

vs., *I always end up hating myself after I eat like this. Why isn't that enough to make me stop wanting to do it??*

It's worth noting that while the emotional brain is not motivated by future results, it is the emotional brain that will experience them when the time comes. That's where you experience the suffering created by short-sighted, impulsive choices.

It is also where you bask in victory and contentment when things turn out well.

Because of the limitations described above, though, the emotional brain can't prioritize future results when making decisions; in a way, it can't see where it's going. Only the cortex can fully comprehend the future, so only the cortex can determine which choices will make the emotional brain the happiest both now *and* in the future.

It Develops Strong Biases

When you have found something enjoyable, that item or experience gets filed in the "like it and want more of it" category, perhaps intensely so. You'll give that experience the benefit of the doubt going forward, classifying it as a good thing because you enjoyed it in the past.

Because it's nice to figure something out and not have to decide about it again, you'll want to keep that mindset. You will, therefore, tend to minimize, rationalize, deny, or simply ignore new evidence that contradicts your initial evaluation.

Consider what happens once you've identified a favorite food, for example. Let's say this food makes you all happy just thinking about it, and you get it as much as you possibly can. Now you find out that this favorite food has some ingredients you find worrisome. Logically, you'd walk away, but this isn't logical. You love the food, so you reassure yourself with rationalizations like, "They wouldn't sell it if it was bad for us," or "I eat a lot of other things that are healthier so it all balances out," or "This is just normal--everybody eats this."

If you heard about the same questionable ingredients in a food you hadn't yet tried, you might feel just fine passing it up. Since it's a food you already love, however, the mental contortions begin. You keep the food in your life and just try a little harder not to think about it. Feelings overpower facts.[1]

How about when you begin to notice that whenever you have certain much-loved foods, you usually end up stuffed, miserable, and hating yourself afterward? Logically, you'd easily walk away from anything that predictably makes you feel miserable and loathsome. Who wouldn't? In this case, *you* wouldn't. Your emotional brain has fixated on these foods as something it wants, based strictly on how enjoyable you hope the foods will be while you're eating them. You'll be hard pressed to come up with enough evidence to get your emotional brain to reconsider this position because again, feelings overpower facts.

The emotional brain's tendency to adopt stubborn biases shows up in many ways above and beyond food issues.[2] Addiction, for example, has to do in part with the emotional brain categorizing something as very desirable, then doggedly pursuing it even in the absence of the expected reward. In other words, you're doing something that's not giving you all you were hoping for, but you feel compelled to keep at it because it really seems like the reward *should* come if you just try hard enough.

The emotional brain will cling to an established bias like this in the face of many, many experiences that fail to bear it out. The tendency is to keep believing rather than destroying that particular mental structure and building something new. This is why we keep turning to food despite ourselves.

Phobias, on the other hand, are in part about the emotional brain categorizing something as a threat, and then doggedly avoiding it even in the absence of the expected harm. The emotional brain will cling to the fear despite things repeatedly turning out just fine, as feelings overrule facts yet again.

Aversions are far less intense than phobias, but can be another example of the emotional brain categorizing something negatively despite information that suggests otherwise.

Many people feel resistant to the idea of nutritious food and regular exercise, for instance, despite the fact that both routinely create enjoyable results. In this case, the emotional brain is convinced that these practices are burdensome rather than rewarding simply because the rewards don't come quickly enough and worse, because some effort is required up front. The emotional brain maintains this bias despite experience to the contrary that with just a little more time, these choices create much more happiness and satisfaction than do most other alternatives.

It Has a *Long* Memory

The emotional brain usually prefers the familiar—"the devil you know"—to the unknown, even if the familiar has obvious drawbacks. This is why you may feel resistant to trying healthier patterns even though you know you need them—you resist them because they are different. It is also why you may abandon those patterns at some future point even if they've been working well for you—some part of you yearns to just relax back into the familiar, despite the fact that it caused the problems that spurred you into change in the first place. A brief glimpse into nervous system function will explain why we have these tendencies.

Whenever you think or do anything, it is made possible by the transmission of electrical signals in your nervous system. These signals move from one nerve cell (neuron) to the next, activating the bodily systems necessary to execute whatever action you have decided to take.

Take the same action repeatedly, and the signal will begin to follow the same cell-to-cell path it traveled previously, establishing a neural pathway that will continue to be used for future repetitions of the same action.

Much like a footpath in the woods that becomes easier to find with repeated use, neural pathways become more robust with practice.[3] The stronger the neural pathway, the more easily and efficiently you can perform that particular action. This is why practice makes perfect, but it's also why old habits die hard.

Your overeating patterns have been practiced thousands of times over many years, creating neural superhighways to enable their operation.

When you go on to create new neural pathways for more fulfilling patterns, the old pathways fall into disuse, but don't disappear. The old pathways remain—well-built but inactive—right alongside the newer ones which support better outcomes, but which are still under construction.

In day-to-day life, this means that when you stop intentionally choosing the newer path, you'll automatically default back to the old one that you know so well.

You can do this so smoothly that you don't even realize it, perhaps "finding" yourself doing something like eating out of a bag of cookies, pulling up to a drive-through, or finishing the kids' leftovers. The shift into the old pattern can be *that* seamless, and it happens in an instant.

You may dream of a time when you can completely forget about the old, painful days of the addiction but the truth is that the neural pathways for it will always remain in place. This is why the risk of relapse generally lasts to some degree for a lifetime. You should exercise extreme caution whenever you notice yourself thinking something like, *I should be able to do this safely <u>now</u>.*

This is not to say that all you have to look forward to is struggling through the remainder of your life, one white-knuckled day at a time. Those new neural pathways, if you've built them to the right places, will actually enable you to calm down and enjoy your life more than ever before.

Nor is it the case that perfect performance is necessary for you to succeed. Momentary lapses are to be expected, but should also be taken seriously. A lapse—any behavior that you didn't plan on, couldn't control, or ultimately made you at all unhappy—is a serious warning that if you're not more cautious going forward, things are likely to get worse.

A lapse with food compares to driving a car and wandering out of your lane until you hit the rumble strips along the edge. Nothing truly bad happens, but you've been put on notice that disaster got closer than usual. Ignore the warning at your own risk.

You're likely to have lapses—hopefully, mostly small ones—for the rest of your life. Just heed them as the warning signs that they are and learn as much as you can from them. Properly examined, each one makes you stronger. Over time, you'll have them less often and recover from them more quickly, but odds are that they'll still pop up periodically. The best response is to just keep learning and moving forward.

It is Poorly Matched to Today's World

There is a profound difference between what enhances survival in the wild and what enhances it in modern life. As a result, our wellbeing is now threatened by the same behavioral tendencies that have protected us for most of our history.

Our preference for sweets is a perfect example—it works out well in the wild, leading us to essential nutrients. In the modern world, however, that same taste preference leads us to overindulgence in products that accelerate numerous disease and addictive processes.

The dilemma is how to channel the power of the emotional brain so that it can once again drive positive outcomes rather than harmful ones, despite being in an unnatural environment that constantly supplies it with misinformation.

This is an easier task to face when you remember what the emotional brain does for you, despite its unique quirks and vulnerabilities.

It is Still Why Life is Worth Living

Have you ever loved someone or felt the warmth of knowing someone loves you? Do you have a hobby or interest that you look forward to doing, which engages you so much that you lose track of time while you're doing it? Have you ever felt the thrill of an unexpected and wonderful surprise? Have you ever felt an upwelling of confidence from overcoming a challenge you weren't sure you could manage? Have you ever had a moment which felt absolutely perfect?

These experiences and all like them come to you courtesy of your emotional brain, because it is where your feelings develop. It's not simply a source of joy and happiness, of course; all of the pain in life happens there too, including the guilt, shame and regret of uncontrolled overeating.

Many people, upon learning that a specific part of the brain drives their compulsive eating, express an urgent desire to have that part surgically removed. Even if that were possible, it would mean that you'd never again have any of the feelings that make for a fully dimensional life. Imagine a life in which everything feels like nothing—do you really want that?

The task, then, is to appreciate what your emotional brain makes possible for you while learning to use it and take care of it more effectively, based on the somewhat odd requirements of today's world. When you do, you'll find that your emotional brain will be the source of more peace, joy, and true contentment than ever before.

Chapter 10
Unexpected Hazards of Modern Life

Modern life offers an abundance of opportunities of many kinds, which actually poses a serious challenge to the emotional brain. When you understand how this works, you can set up your life to be much simpler, calmer, more satisfying, and more enjoyable.

The Problem of Too Much

The emotional brain is geared toward rapid judgement of the elements in its world, and rapid action based on that judgement. In a world of scarce resources and limited opportunities, the "get what you can whenever you can get it" system works well. There is little need for behavioral self-regulation in nature simply because there is so little opportunity for excess of any kind.

This is not to say we are incapable of self-regulation. The problem is that our capacity for it does not reside in the emotional brain, which happens to have the greatest immediate power in how decisions get made.

Most of us now have constant access to hyperpalatable food. The emotional brain reacts to this abundance just as it would to the limited opportunities for which it is adapted: by trying to have it all. It is very *un*natural to have food available and have the physical ability to eat more of it, yet choose to stop eating. The emotional brain simply does not operate this way.

Food is not the only field on which this problem plays out. Given the emotional brain's preference for quick reward and for exploiting immediate opportunities in general, it's not hard to see how abundance and easy opportunity of any kind has the potential to take a wrong turn.

Consider some other everyday indulgences that carry a known risk of addiction: alcohol use, drug use, smoking, sex, spending, gambling, and online activities. It's certainly possible to pursue any of these without lapsing into self-destructiveness and many people do, but a great many also fail in the attempt. Loss of personal control in such instances shows you an emotional brain unintentionally self-destructing as it applies the "get all you can" strategy to a situation in which it is possible to get too much. "Enough" is not an emotional brain concept. The emotional brain, left to its own devices, is unable to stop until the negative consequences of excess make it too painful to continue, or until there is simply no more opportunity.

The Powerful, Defenseless Emotional Brain

The cortex can easily provide the self-regulation that makes it possible for the emotional brain to live happily and healthily in a world of too much.

The problem is that the emotional brain is intensely activated by opportunity, and can be triggered into an internal power grab that locks out the cortex. If this happens, the emotional brain is left unguided where it can't protect itself. Chaos, frustration, and regret are the predictable result.

The need for frequent, deliberate self-management is quite new to us as a species, yet its importance is intensifying more with each passing year. The requirement for it now is dramatically higher than it was just 40 to 50 years ago, let alone for all of human history prior to that. It is perhaps understandable that it's been hard for most of us to keep up with what it takes to survive in our very different world of the present.

At the time of this writing, reality TV is a well-established genre, including a subset devoted to survival in the wild with minimal support. These programs show how valuable our basic drives still are once we're back in a setting that fits them. Cast members do exactly what we all *want* to do: they eat everything they can find and rest whenever they can. Their setting involves few opportunities for food and rest, so this promotes survival.

In our setting with endless opportunity for both, the same choices are ruining millions of lives.

Self-Management for Life

It is vital to understand the mismatch between how our brains work and what is required by the conditions in which we now live. Our core survival drives, left unchecked in conditions of overabundance, result in behavior that promotes self-destruction rather than survival.

We are well-equipped to handle this mismatch as long as we can keep the cortex engaged. So, how can we do that? The answer is *not* in strengthening the cortex so that it can get better at controlling the impulsive emotional brain, because that isn't possible.

What *does* work is to keep the emotional brain calm enough to be receptive to higher-level strategies. It is when the emotional brain becomes reactive—as with excitement, anticipation, depression, anxiety, or anger—that it can start to override the cortex. This is why no amount of logic seems sufficient to overcome an intense desire to eat.

As long as you continue to live in an environment of easy excess, it will be necessary to remain conscious and intentional about food in your life. This is not a punishment or a burden—it is simply a factual requirement of how we now live. Your emotional brain will always be on hot standby, ready to spring into action with those old drives if it is triggered too much. The only solution is to minimize how much that happens.

Chapter 11
The Key to Living Well in Today's World

Back in Chapter 8, our animal companions helped us to see the general characteristics and vulnerabilities of the emotional brain. This was possible because compared to us, they (bless their hearts) don't have much of a cortex in place to obstruct the view.

We have capacities for thought, understanding, learning, and problem-solving that they lack, so we use our much larger and more able cortex on their behalf. We do this because it's obvious that there are aspects of their world they can't comprehend, and that we need to make some extra efforts to assure their safety.

There's not much in the wild that compares with getting burned on a hot stovetop or hit by a car, for example, so our pets lack the instincts that would enable them avoid such hazards. We compensate for this by doing our best to keep them out of situations we know they can't accurately assess for potential danger. Because "poison" is not a concept they can grasp, we have to assure they have no access to antifreeze, household chemicals, and any number of "people foods" that they find highly attractive, but which could harm them.

Because our pets benefit from the protection made possible by our cortex, they are generally able to thrive despite living in close proximity to all manner of risks they will never understand.

We Need to Protect *Our* Emotional Brain, Too
Our own emotional brain needs the protection of our cortex just as surely as our pets do, and for the same reason. We are predisposed toward unintentional self-harm in the face of modern challenges we are not wired to handle, especially that of sustained abundance. Fortunately, watching out for ourselves in the face of risk is something we're already very good at. We do it all the time.

Have you ever worn a helmet for any reason? Ear protection? Gloves? Heavier clothing on a cold day? Rain gear on a wet day?

Do you look both ways before crossing a roadway?

41

Do you exercise extra care when handling sharp objects?

Do you ever lock your house or car?

You've probably done all of these things and many more like them. You take actions like these continually, effortlessly, and without resentment. You do this because it is natural to assess your environment for potential problems, then to address them in ways that assure your continued safety, security and comfort.

We don't think twice about protecting our eyes, ears, hands, feet, or even our belongings. We just accept it as part of living and work it into our routines. The emotional brain is simply one more item to include on the lengthy list of things that are worth watching out for.

The Two Yous in Conflict

It has long been recognized that we deal with conflicting energies or voices within ourselves, commonly expressed in ways similar to these:

Part of me says to do it but another part says not to.

I know in my head that this makes no sense, but my heart really wants it.

I've got an angel on one shoulder and a devil on the other.

You may now start to see that this kind of conflict can be traced back to the emotional brain and the cortex.[1] These two parts of the brain see the world through very different lenses, applying radically different priorities to decision-making. They have something of a relationship and if you've been moved to read this book, it's probably a difficult one.

If that's the case, you probably look at your emotional brain as an unruly troublemaker that does stupid, destructive things. You may sometimes feel a desperate need to control or restrain it so that it won't destroy everything and ruin your life.

You may see your cortex, on the other hand, as the fun police demanding a barren existence devoid of pleasures, all in the name of *health*. Such a life would hardly be worth living so naturally, you resist.

Many people with overeating issues have low self-esteem, with a relationship between the emotional brain and cortex as described above. If that's the way it is inside, there's not much left to feel good about. The chronic emotional pain caused by this creates a need for comfort and relief, which triggers more eating. The vicious cycle continues.

These two parts of you have ended up set against each other due to the oddities of modern life, but it doesn't have to be that way. Even in our current circumstances, it is possible to combine the adaptive capacity of your cortex with the power and passion of your emotional brain, getting the best of both worlds while keeping both happy.

When you do that, you get calm, confident self-esteem in addition to creating a life that is full, effective, and deeply satisfying.

The Two Yous at Peace

A good relationship between the emotional brain and the cortex allows the two to pull together toward the same goals rather than working at cross purposes. No part of you gets ignored or marginalized, so there are no more internal power struggles. Such power struggles are well worth avoiding because they are counterproductive and draining, and they only end when one part of *you* loses.

A healthier process will take care of you as a whole, rather than attempting to sacrifice one part of the system for the intended benefit of the rest.

In this calmer, happier internal relationship, the emotional brain gets the lead role, because it has to. It has the most power due to housing basic survival drives, but is also where you feel secondary needs like meaning, passion, belonging, fun, fulfillment, comfort, and peace.

The problem is that your emotional brain lacks the capacity to develop effective strategies for achieving these benefits in the modern world.

Left to its own devices, it tends to come up with ideas like eating half a pie or staying online for hours on end. Such choices may seem appealing up front, but often end in feelings of apathy, depression, and even self-loathing, all felt by the same emotional brain that was just seeking comfort in the first place. What the emotional brain desperately needs for real happiness is a good guidance system. Enter the cortex.

Ideally, the cortex works in service to the emotional brain, though many people try to use it as a bullying supervisor instead. This is doomed to failure given the emotional brain's built-in power advantage. Rather than being a supervisor to the emotional brain, the cortex is more like the hired help, with a job description that involves roles like personal assistant, compassionate guide, caretaker, and creative problem-solver.

The cortex has many talents the emotional brain lacks, starting with its ability to assess the modern environment more accurately. It can learn more from the past and see further into the future. It can generate more alternatives for meeting a need in the moment, and is better at figuring out which ones are likely to create the best payoffs.

It can see the potential for hazards and steer around them altogether, or work at damage control when that is required. It can turn on a dime to account for changing conditions, opportunities and risks, to chart the most rewarding probable course of action for the emotional brain.

The cortex can't force the emotional brain to accept any of this goodness, however, because for all its impressive capabilities, it really *is* subservient to the emotional brain.

You experience this each time you try to force yourself to do something that you know is a good idea, but which you really don't want to do. You feel great resistance inside and if you are able to push past it at all, you will likely only manage it temporarily. Eventually, what you want the most will rule the day, despite how much you may know better.

Another item in the cortex's job description then, is to remember its place in the power hierarchy, which is at the bottom. From there, the cortex's most effective position is that of compassionate and concerned advisor, dedicated to the authentic and lasting happiness of the emotional brain.

The unguided emotional brain will fall for false or fleeting happiness almost every time but the cortex won't; it can work instead to persuade the emotional brain toward the choices that create the most substantial and lasting enjoyment.

When the cortex is geared toward working *for* the emotional brain rather than trying to subdue it, the emotional brain becomes more open to considering alternatives. This is because we relate to our own self-talk the same way we do to input from anyone else. We tend to listen more when we're convinced the speaker is a friendly ally.

Conversely, if someone is yelling at us and bullying us, it doesn't matter how much sense they might happen to be making—we will defensively shut them out and not hear what they're trying to say. So it is with the emotional brain and the cortex, which means that the final entry on the cortex's job description is to be kind, always. Be caring, be supportive, be protective, and be respectful with yourself as you use your cortex to influence your emotional brain toward the choices that create the best life you can possibly have.

Your cortex is well-equipped for these duties once you realize you are better off using it this way. Like everything else, you'll get better at it with practice. The beauty of it is that even as you make mistakes along the way while learning to use your cortex more effectively, you'll still be getting better results than if you just left your emotional brain to blunder about on its own.

When you use your cortex to meet your emotional brain's needs as effectively as possible, you will finally discover real emotional peace. This is not the illusion of peace you get from succumbing to the overwhelming urge to eat—all you're really experiencing then is a temporary ceasefire in your head since that particular battle has been decided. Using your brain in a cooperative, coordinated fashion creates real peace, real balance, and real comfort.

Every part of you wins in this scenario. The cortex is kept busy with the creative and productive work at which it excels, the emotional brain gets more reliable fulfillment of its core needs, and the body gets better care as a result. Improving physical and emotional health create increasing rewards to the emotional brain, creating a positive feedback loop to replace the vicious cycle of the past.

The Power of Inner Unity

The secret to personal peace is a safe and happy emotional brain, and the secret to *that* is a consistently engaged cortex. Keep the two working together, and you will find yourself much more balanced with food, but also more generally effective in life. You will create better results, thus building greater confidence. You will experience greater creativity and motivation. You will tackle challenges with greater ease. Life will become more interesting and more enjoyable.

At its most focused, this is the state you've perhaps heard referred to as flow, being in the zone, or as peak performance. Regardless of the language, such moments are among the high points in life. As you get better at using your brain in a unified way, you'll get more of those moments than ever before.

You might doubt your potential for this level of effectiveness when you feel like a chronic failure with food. The fact is that food presents one of the greatest challenges to this kind of unified operation, and for the simplest of reasons. Adequate nourishment is a survival imperative, so our food-related drives are among the most intense that we have. These powerful drives are readily activated, and we now have to manage them in an atmosphere of near-constant opportunity. This is why we can be so accomplished, so competent, and so wise in other areas of our lives, yet fall apart over and over again when it comes to food.

Fortunately, this predicament can be managed once you are prepared for the challenges you are most likely to encounter along the way.

Part Three

Common Psychological Hurdles on the Path Toward Change

Chapter 12
The Fallacy of Normal

The core desire expressed to me by many overeaters is "to just be able to eat like a normal person," but that raises the question of what they are assuming to be normal. Most seem to imagine that it means maintaining easy self-control despite chronic exposure to highly triggering foods. They remain convinced of this despite the fact that they rarely see it practiced in the world around them.

I ask each client whom they know in any context, who demonstrates the comfort and self-control with food that they hope to achieve. About half the time, the answer to the question is "no one." The next most common response is to be able to name only one person. Fewer than 10% of my clients can identify two or more people—out of everyone they know in every area of their lives—who have the self-control with food that they assume normal people have.

It's not clear where all the presumed normal people might be when it's so hard to find many who fit the description.

It might be easier to abandon the word *normal* altogether and stick with more objective descriptions of what people are actually doing. Toward that end, I can offer information I have gathered from approximately 3,000 detailed clinical assessments I've conducted over the years.

Nearly 1,000 of these clients came to me specifically for therapy related to overeating, while the remaining 2,000 sought treatment for other issues like depression, marital problems, grief, or any number of other general dilemmas that tend to lead people to therapy. Many of those other 2,000 clients who came in for non-eating issues were, in fact, overeaters (as the statistics would suggest), but happened to seek therapy for something else. The remainder actually weren't overeaters, which now makes them a handy comparison group.

I have found that most people tend to fit into one of three general categories regarding their eating and general self-care practices at any given time: overeaters, dieters, and people who are living in balance with food.

Overeaters

Many overeaters rely a lot on food prepared by others in order to get through their weeks. They eat out, bring food in, or have it delivered on a regular basis.

Cooking, when it happens, often involves the use of processed products designed to make the meal easier to prepare. Many overeaters no longer know very much about cooking and see it as a poor use of their limited time. Some, though, do cook at home regularly, using plenty of fresh, whole ingredients; though many of their meals are of high quality, they remain subject to other pitfalls that ultimately undermine their sense of self-control.

Overeaters often eat with little discernible pattern; sometimes they graze all day but sometimes they go many hours with no food, followed by binge eating when they have the opportunity. Their portion sizes are usually far in excess of what is required to meet their bodies' fuel needs.

Most prioritize food that is easy, economical, and enjoyable. They address their health and weight concerns by purchasing products specially formulated to be low fat, low sugar, low calorie, gluten-free, high protein, high fiber, vitamin-enriched, or possessing whatever other characteristic they believe to be helpful.

They drink many prepared beverages, heavily biased toward regular soda, diet soda, and specialty coffee products.[1] Most drink water infrequently if at all; when they do, it is usually only when nothing tastier is readily available.

They exercise little, if at all, even when they have the physical ability to do so. Their hobbies and work both tend to be sedentary, so there's not much reason for them to move beyond the basic need to change location periodically through the day.

They organize their socializing around food, rarely if ever getting together with friends or family to share any activity other than eating, conversation, and perhaps a viewed sporting event or movie.

Dieters

Unlike overeaters, dieters prepare a lot of food at home. Depending on the diet, this may be mostly whole food that is home-cooked, or it may involve plan-specific foods that are simply heated up when needed. Home food preparation is accepted as a necessary part of dieting, though not necessarily embraced as an ongoing way of life beyond the diet. Any special foods or supplements that are required are purchased from the business that promotes the diet.

Dieters eat quantities and on a structured schedule as prescribed by the diet. Their priority is weight loss, and their focus is on careful adherence to the procedures specific to the diet they have chosen. These patterns are usually seen as a temporary necessity rather than as the beginning of a new way of life, and are generally followed only as long as the person considers themselves to be "on the diet."

Their core beverages are water, diet soda, plain coffees or teas, and/or special drinks designed as part of the diet plan. These beverage choices are generally not maintained for long once the diet is finished or abandoned.

Most exercise regularly as part of the diet plan, except for those whose plans promise weight loss without exercise. Those who exercise as part of the diet usually discontinue soon after they stop dieting.

Dieters get together with friends and family to share food, but may tend to do so less while dieting so that they can stay on course. They sometimes bring their own food to such events since what they need to eat is usually different from that which will be served to the group. Most of them eventually revert to their old socializing patterns and activities once they are off the diet.

Balanced Eaters

Balanced eaters make most of their meals at home, using mostly whole food ingredients. They may include some prepared or processed foods, but do not consider those items to be staples.

They accept home food preparation as essential to maintaining the level of health that they want so it's not a matter of debate—they just do it. If they're not very good at it, they keep the recipes very simple, but they keep cooking.

Their eating has a fairly regular rhythm to it from one day to the next, organized largely around eating when hungry and stopping when satisfied. Their portion sizes are large enough for pleasurable eating and for meeting nutritional needs, but not large enough to support excess weight. Their priority is to have food that is enjoyable today and which also supports strong health for the future.

Their core beverage is water, supplemented by minimally adulterated teas and coffees. Sodas are consumed rarely, if at all.

They tend to be generally active people, with many exercising regularly or even daily. As with cooking, they accept a certain amount of physical activity as an essential factor for the life they want; they prioritize around it, assuring that time is kept available for it.

Their social activities with friends and families often include food, but the companionship and other shared activities (games, sports, events, walks, visits to local attractions, etc.) are the main point of getting together.

How Life Experiences Compare

If you look carefully at the groups above, you'll notice there are really only *two* groups. There are overeaters who bounce back and forth between dieting and giving up, and balanced eaters who just keep living the same way year after year. Comparing these groups reveals fascinating differences in what their lives are like.

Food Temptation

Overeaters hear the call of especially tempting food a lot of the time and usually give in to it, often feeling quietly guilty about doing so. They manage to resist it sometimes, but usually find this difficult and disappointing. They occasionally find actual respite from temptation in dieting, as they are able to accept such food as temporarily off limits. Unfortunately, this does not last.

Many people believe that balanced eaters are naturally unfazed by tempting foods or are simply strong enough to resist them, but this is true of only a few. Most would feel the same urges that overeaters do— they simply organize their lives so that they don't have to deal with it that much. Wrestling with temptation then, is something nearly exclusive to overeaters not because they are more vulnerable to it, but because they are more exposed to it.

Feelings of Physical and Emotional Wellness

Overeaters usually feel "okay" for the most part, though often with varying signs of sluggishness or depression; they are usually surprised by how much better they feel while dieting. Balanced eaters are accustomed to feeling energetic, clear, strong, and enthusiastic most of the time.

Immune System Function

While colds and other opportunistic infections may seem like an inevitable part of life, the reality is that they are experienced to a far greater degree by those with poor nutrition and sedentary habits.

Most of the high-calorie foods favored by overeaters are inflammation-producing foods which cause the immune system to work harder than it otherwise would. Because the immune system is constantly dealing with diet-related inflammation, it has less remaining capacity for dealing with invasive bacteria and viruses.[2]

Someone with a poor diet is therefore more vulnerable not only to opportunistic infections like colds and influenza, but also to more chronic inflammatory conditions like vascular disease and diabetes. In contrast, the diets of balanced eaters naturally tend toward *anti-inflammatory* foods. This leaves their immune systems more fully charged, which reduces their vulnerability to both passing infections and chronic disease.

An additional advantage enjoyed by balanced eaters is the fact that they tend to engage in vigorous activity on a regular basis. One of the ways that your body fights infection when you become ill is to raise its temperature, which you might notice as a fever. This is bad news for many of the microbes that may try to take over your system because when they become too warm, they die. Fighting off an illness is good, but what if you could sometimes prevent it from happening in the first place?

When balanced eaters regularly exercise, work, or play hard enough to raise their body temperature a bit, the warmer internal environment kills off some microbes before they've taken enough of a hold to start creating symptoms. The body in such cases has killed off the invaders so quickly that as far as you know, nothing has happened at all.[3] It's not a foolproof system because balanced eaters certainly do get sick sometimes, but not often.

Aches and Pains

Overeaters commonly have numerous aches and pains directly traceable to the effects of their inflammation-producing diet[4] and inactivity, though they often notice some improvement while dieting and moving more. Balanced eaters are generally pain-free except for injuries and the normal deterioration of advancing age, and even those are easier for them than they are for overeaters.

Gastrointestinal Function

Many overeaters suffer chronic constipation due to their low-fiber, low-quality diet, sedentary lifestyle, and the side effects of medications they may require for control of hypertension[5] or depression.[6] While overeaters may come to accept constipation as an inevitable part of life, it is virtually unknown to balanced eaters since they tend to stay well-hydrated, well-fed, physically active, and to need few if any medications.

Emotional Experience

Overeaters live with a lot of subtle unrest. They feel like they probably should be doing healthier things, but fear that change would be too hard and might not be worth the trouble. When dieting, they tend to feel resentful about what they "have to do" even as they notice that it makes them feel physically better. Balanced eaters feel good and are determined to stay that way; they find it baffling that overeaters are willing to put up with living the way they do.

Weight

Most overeaters experience a gradual, lifelong increase in their average weight. Many of them will experience large spikes along the way as they drop weight while dieting, later regaining and adding to it in the rebound. Even during the times when they believe their weight to be stable, they consider it normal to vary within as much as a 10-20 pound range. Balanced eaters, by contrast, experience minimal daily variation while remaining at the same or nearly the same average weight throughout their lives. Some will put on a bit more in their senior years, but will still remain far leaner than their peers who overeat.

Aging

Nobody escapes age-related decline, but for overeaters, it comes earlier and with greater impact. As overeaters in retirement are becoming steadily more confined by poor health and limited mobility, most balanced eaters are remaining more active, interested, and involved.

The difference between an "old 70" and a "young 70" in today's world, for example, is often the difference between an overeater and a balanced eater. It is in the later years that the cruelest irony of overeating becomes most visible, as the weight and the medical problems it causes result in physical limitations that reduce other options for enjoying life.

As the other options are gradually lost, the eating that took them away becomes one of the few things left to do at all, making it increasingly important even as it continues to erode remaining quality of life. The worse it is, the worse it gets.

Beyond "Normal"

The reality for most people in industrialized societies today is to struggle with food, to suffer unwanted consequences, and to continue doing so despite knowing better. This is obviously not what anyone wants, and we don't have to settle for it.

What people clearly *do* want is to be able just to relax in life, not having to make complex decisions about eating or health all the time, focusing instead on the business or pleasure of each day as it comes, including easy enjoyment of the food along the way.

It will serve you well to abandon the idea of an idealized normal that does not exist, so you can focus instead on what works for you, what makes you stronger and happier, and what helps you to create the life you really want.

Chapter 13
All-or-Nothing Thinking

All-or-nothing thinking is quite common in the general population and nearly universal among overeaters in their approach to food, weight, and health. It tells you that once you've eaten a cookie, you might as well polish off the rest because you've blown it now anyway. It also tells you that if you don't have time for a complete workout, there's no point in doing anything at all.

This polarized style of thinking has now led you to eat a whole bag of cookies and skip your workout, when you might otherwise have eaten a couple of cookies and exercised as much as you could. The latter outcome would clearly be far superior, yet would be judged as a failure because it was not perfect.

Such is the warped perspective that all-or-nothing thinking creates, devaluing worthwhile efforts while demanding a level of performance that no one can maintain 100% of the time. Thinking this way generates failure and hopelessness rather than supporting health and wellbeing. It oversimplifies your efforts into a binary framework in which you're either doing well or you're not, with no value given to honest efforts or improved outcomes that fall short of the imagined ideal.

The reality is that your performance doesn't have to be perfect, but it does need to be good enough to move you closer to the life you want, one step at a time. That's the only measure of your efforts that means anything.

If, from one month to the next, you can see that you're gradually making higher quality decisions for yourself with greater consistency, you're doing fine. If you're not seeing that, it means you need to adjust your approach. You'll do better on some days than on others, but the most important thing is that you keep doing the best you can through good days and bad. In the end, it is persistence rather than perfection that will get you what you want.

Would you like a life in which you could have most of what you want and need, most of the time? When you move all-or-nothing thinking out of the way, that opens up lots of room in which "most" can happen. When you focus on maintaining a strong effort and appreciating better outcomes rather than demanding perfect ones, you will find that such a life is easier to achieve than you ever imagined.

Chapter 14
Fear of Getting Nutrition Wrong

Many of us are paralyzed into inaction when we are afraid of doing something wrong, partly because nobody likes being wrong and partly out of fear of making mistakes that could matter. Given the volume of nutritional advice now available—much of it contradictory—many people have stopped even trying to get it right, deferring instead to the foods that are the easiest or most fun.

This strategy reduces stress by ending the tiring internal debate in any given moment. It also replaces the hard job of figuring out the best foods with the easy job of choosing the most enjoyable ones. The downside is that it results in poor nutrition, compromised health, and lost quality of life.

This process of agonizing over what and how to eat is specific to life in the developed world, where the sheer volume of choices makes nutrition seem complex and perhaps beyond the understanding of most ordinary people.

It may be useful to remember that all animals come wired with the tendencies that they need in order to survive. Given adequate access to food, all will manage to feed themselves properly without expert intervention, as humans have for many thousands of years.

Nutrition Made Simple
Imagine for a moment that you're living in the wilderness, without the tools or foods and beverages of the developed world. Since you're an omnivore, your body is adapted to the digestion of most plants or animals you can find, but you usually don't have many decisions to make about what to eat. You just get whatever you can, hoping to avoid anything toxic along the way.

The matter of what to drink is easily settled because water is the only choice you generally have. You might have access to some particularly juicy fruit or find some vegetation that works well for tea but water will tend to be your core beverage.

Next, there's the question of how to feed yourself in an environment where physical safety is paramount. Vegetation of some kind is your best bet simply because that's what's easiest, safest, and most plentiful. Vegetation can't run away, doesn't fight back, and is practically everywhere, so it's your most reliable go-to food source.

Your next most available choice would probably be things like bugs, grubs, worms, and snails which, though they lack a certain aesthetic appeal, would be an important and generally available source of calories and protein. Non-poisonous frogs, lizards and snakes would be a considerable improvement when you could safely catch them. You'd probably welcome the chance to raid the occasional bird's nest of eggs when possible.

Next up would likely be fish. They're challenging to catch, but most of the fish you can find are not going to represent a direct threat. You may well injure yourself in the act of fishing, but are unlikely to be wounded by your prey.

Small game comes at the next level of risk. You won't usually get as much as you'd like because most small creatures are quick and hard to take by surprise. There's also the disadvantage that they fight back. Getting clawed or bitten can be death in the wild, so you only go after mammals when you really must. Bigger game is a wonderful thing, but the risks associated with bagging it are much, much greater. You get serious meat when you can but it's just too dangerous and unreliable a food source to be a core part of your diet.

Keeping Nutrition Simple in Modern Life
The life described above may not sound inviting, but it does describe the dietary conditions to which our bodies have adapted over most of human history. There's a reason our health professionals often tell us to drink more water and eat a plant-based diet with much less emphasis on meat. The closer we get to the diet that has molded our systems for thousands of years, the healthier, more energetic, and longer-lived we tend to be.

The dietary patterns we would have in the wild serve as a good benchmark for the choices that make the most sense for us in the lives we actually lead. It takes a little more effort and investment than grabbing bags of snacks or getting dinner from the drive-through, but at least it's simple as long as you base your diet primarily on real, whole food rather than on manufactured products.

People who stock their kitchens and pantries with this in mind tend to keep fresh and frozen produce on hand at all times. They use beans and lentils in a variety of recipes and salads, as an easy and economical source of plant-based protein and fiber. They may use nuts and seeds as snacks and in recipes, though sparingly, due to the higher calorie content.

Those who eat lean meats, poultry and seafood buy them fresh or frozen to cook at home, rather than using prepared entrees that involve coatings, sauces, and fillers. Many such people keep eggs on hand as a convenient, easily prepared source of protein. They choose breads, cereals and pastas that are made from whole grains.[1] They tend toward low-fat dairy products, keeping a careful eye on labels for additives they wish to avoid, especially added sugars. Water, tea, and coffee tend to be their beverages of choice.

Since most of us are likely to continue using some manufactured food products in our homes, it is important to learn how to select the most nutritionally useful among them. While some manufactured products include meaningful amounts of whole food, others include only trace amounts of it for marketing purposes.

A quick way to assess such products is to consider which of them could theoretically be reproduced in a home kitchen by a knowledgeable cook using ingredients available from a neighborhood grocery store. Products failing this test may be of questionable food value.

All You Really Need to Know

Your imagined life in the wild says it all: drink mostly water and eat a varied, plant-based diet. If you eat meat, make sure it's primarily lean meat and that you use it as a supplement rather than as the foundation of your diet, a change that many in the industrialized world will struggle to accept. You may at least be relieved to know that we can get all the nutrients we need without resorting to the bugs, worms, and such which were a matter of necessity for so many of our ancestors, and which remain so for many people in the developing parts of the world today.

Barring individual medical conditions that dictate otherwise, that's all there is to it.

Beware the all-or-nothing thinking (Chapter 13) that suggests you must eat *exactly* this way or you're not doing enough. This is an ideal that would indeed provide optimal nutritional support for your body, so if and when you really want to do that, you'll know how. Until then, if you use the ideal as something to gradually move toward over time, your personal nutrition will improve with each step closer to it that you take.

Chapter 15
Critical Misperceptions

The emotional brain makes snap judgments based on immediate impressions, but modern life offers many initial impressions that are misleading. As a result, the emotional brain can lock onto ideas or decisions that are based on faulty information, resulting in behaviors that are unintentionally self-destructive. In a life that is fast-paced and full of distractions, it can be hard to slow down and focus enough to see why you repeatedly make choices you later regret.

Misdefining Food

When I conduct community education seminars on the issue of overeating, the easiest way to help participants see the perceptual distortions of the emotional brain is to provide an opportunity for those distortions to be experienced in real time.

When I ask what they find most rewarding to eat, most people will identify dessert or snack items. When asked what they find least rewarding to eat, most people will immediately reply, "'Vegetables!" I then ask them some questions about how it works when their eating involves a lot of the treat foods they've now defined as rewarding:

"How do you tend to feel physically?"

"How is your mood affected?"

"How is your physical performance affected?"

"How resistant are you to colds and other illnesses?

The light starts to go on for everyone in the group at the same time. They begin to realize that their most cherished foods, after a fleeting moment of pleasure, have a very negative impact on their enjoyment of life.

We then review the same questions about how it works when their eating involves a lot of vegetables, which they have identified as unrewarding. It is an additional moment of clarity for the group when they realize that the much maligned vegetables, upon reflection, reliably improve their enjoyment of life.

Our emotional brain is using the same criterion for food selection that it has always used: whatever is most enjoyable in the moment is the best thing. Until just the last few generations, this worked most of the time.

But we now live surrounded by foods that provide intense sensory pleasure with little nutritional benefit, so the emotional brain is mistakenly pulling hard toward foods that threaten our survival rather than supporting it. Worse yet, the emotional brain is actually rejecting foods that *do* support survival because those foods lack the sheer sensory impact of their artificially enhanced competition.

This stunning, dangerous reversal of priorities is evident whenever someone speaks of real, quality food with disdain, using terms like "diet food," "healthy food," or even "good food" with a sarcastic or dismissive tone. It's amazing that we have learned to casually reject the life-sustaining substances that countless millions have begged, fought and died for throughout human history.

Alternatively, "normal food" is a term usually used in loving reference to desserts, snacks, and take-out meals that are noteworthy for being cheap, easy, and having remarkable sensory punch. They typically do little if anything to support health, and many of them are actually harmful.

Many, though edible and immensely entertaining, technically aren't even food. They may also be referred to as "bad food," but in a manner that implies longing for the forbidden rather than rejection of the mediocre.

It is a cruel irony that the emotional brain has such a powerful bias toward the highly triggering, processed foods that will later cause it such regret, suffering, and even hopelessness.

An individual who struggles with this bias will repeatedly make decisions that trade moments of sensory reward for years of greater physical and emotional misery.

A society of such individuals will teach its children the *opposite* of what they need to know about food in order to thrive, thus ensuring that each new generation will be successively sicker and more disabled at earlier ages. As noted in Chapter 5, this trend is well underway in the U.S. and is being reported with increasing frequency in other developed nations as well.[1]

Misdefining Moderation

Moderation is a simple concept, describing nothing more than the avoidance of extremes—too much or too little—that cause problems. We readily embrace and seek the benefits of moderation, for example, each time we drive.

We don't want to drive so slowly that we waste time, but we don't want to drive so fast that we risk getting a ticket or being in an accident. The speed that captures the best of both worlds—efficient travel time with minimized risk—is a calculation of moderation.

Moderation is made possible by the ability of the cortex to assess multiple variables and determine the balance among them that generates the best total reward.

Maximizing reward is an essential goal of the emotional brain, but it is adapted to the conditions of the wild where it is seldom necessary to balance many variables at once, let alone some that involve the misleading cues that are typical of so many modern foods. The emotional brain is simply not capable of maximizing rewards in the complex environment of the modern world, especially when intensely activated by any primary survival drive; it routinely incurs unintended self-harm when it tries.

I've polled many clients and seminar participants on their gut reaction to moderation, asking them whether they are more likely to feel resentful or grateful about it. The vast majority of people quickly respond that they feel resentful, which is an emotional brain response.

The emotional brain wants all that it can get, so any sense of limitation—no matter how reasonable and beneficial—is quickly judged and rejected.

Gratitude for moderation, on the other hand, shows an engaged cortex. The cortex sees that moderation makes it possible to eat essentially any food you want,[2] and that moderation is the only way in the modern world that you can do so without self-harm. Moderation assures that we will have enough for true enjoyment, but not so much that we're left feeling overstuffed, regretful, or ashamed after the fact.

The problem we have with appreciating moderation has to do with time. Moderation maximizes rewards, which is what the emotional brain wants, but the most substantial of those rewards occur in the future which is beyond the emotional brain's perceptual field.

That future might be as close as five minutes from now when you are relieved (which will happen in your emotional brain, by the way) that you managed to leave the restaurant without ordering dessert. The future is also days, months, or years away, when you will be enjoying (again, in your emotional brain) the better life, stronger health, and greater personal happiness made possible by the moderate choices you've made along the way.

The cortex can easily see how to set up a future the emotional brain will enjoy the most but the emotional brain—where the decision-making power lies—is most strongly motivated by gains in the present, with minimal sense of future cost. Given its thousands of generations of adapting to conditions of scarcity, the emotional brain defines "the right amount" of food in the present as "all you can get," rather than "the amount that you'll enjoy the most with no regrets."

Therefore, it may *feel* like you're losing out for no good reason in the present when you voluntarily take less food than you could, despite the fact that doing so will likely make you happier in the long run. This is why it's so hard to take two cookies and walk away from the rest, for example. In such moments, you may wish that you could eat with more restraint. Later on, you may *really* wish that you had, but at the time, it was just too hard to resist.

Few of us are inherently good at moderation—we're not wired for it because life for many thousands of years did not require it. Then, life in just the past few generations changed so much and so rapidly that we couldn't adapt fast enough to keep up.

As a consequence, we are left with the task of adapting by intention rather than through evolution. We have to, because evolution will take dozens if not hundreds of generations to catch up, and we're on only the third or fourth one so far. If we don't work to save ourselves, the changes we need won't happen in time for us, our kids, our grandkids, or any of our descendants beyond them, for a long, long time.

Intentional adaptation is challenging. It requires us to purposely make choices that make little sense to the emotional brain, given that it can't comprehend how to maximize rewards in the modern world. Fortunately, the cortex can help with this as long as it's kept in the loop.

You can use your cortex to warm your emotional brain up to the idea of moderation with some simple, reality-based questions about concrete past results. For example, if you're having dinner and are feeling drawn to the idea of taking seconds even though you probably don't need any more food, try pausing for a moment to ponder questions like these:

How has my body ended up feeling after doing this in the past?

How have I felt about myself after doing this in the past?

How many times have I done this and been really happy afterward that I did?

How many times have I done this and really wished afterward that I hadn't?

Lingering on the answers and on the feeling-based memories evoked by questions like these can be enough to help the emotional brain sense the real reward of moderation in the present. When you can *feel* the reality of the reward, you become more genuinely interested in choosing it.

In this case, you might feel more able to try something like getting up and walking away for a moment so you can think more clearly. This is a good idea because trying to make these decisions right in front of the food is unreasonably difficult. Your emotional brain at such times is highly triggered by the eating you've just done, the taste remaining in your mouth, the sight and smell of the food in front of you, and the fact that others around you may be continuing to eat.

You can always eat more if you really need to, so you have nothing to lose by pausing to allow time for your emotional brain to calm down and for your cortex to come more actively online. Working from your cortex will enable you to choose food of the type and quantity that you can enjoy in the present, but which you can also feel good about after the fact.

You get the immediate moments of pleasure from the food, followed by hours of satisfaction in knowing you handled yourself well. This is an absolute win-win outcome for the emotional brain, which gets to enjoy feeling content and confident rather than ashamed and in pain.

Moderation is the only way to assure such satisfying outcomes, and only the cortex has that capability. If you're making higher quality food decisions in the present but are feeling resentful and deprived for hours afterward, that simply shows that your strategy needs to be tweaked to better cover the emotional brain's needs. Your cortex can do that, too.

Misdefining Exercise, Part One

I've asked many people for their gut reaction to the idea of exercising. The majority quickly assume a sour facial expression accompanied by an unhappy utterance of some kind. Few people welcome the *idea* of exercise. Their demeanor on the topic generally softens considerably when they consider their personal answers to questions like these, referring to times in the past when they've had more regular physical activity:

"How did you feel physically?"

"How did it affect your mood?"

"How did it affect your energy level?"

"How did you feel about yourself?"

"How often has it happened that you exercised and wished you hadn't?"

"How often has it happened that you didn't exercise but wished you had?"

It's amazing to watch as people quickly morph from a position of, "I hate exercise," to, "Oh right—I actually like what happens when I do it." This happens almost every time.

The initial reaction, of course, comes straight from the emotional brain. Its skills were honed over countless generations in the wild where lots of physical effort is required for survival, and where any energy you have is best conserved for those times when it's really needed.

The emotional brain is primed to value physical action only when an *immediate* benefit is apparent—you need to defend yourself from a predator, seek shelter, forage for dinner, or have an opportunity to do something pleasurable, for example—and to seek rest whenever possible the rest of the time. In a life where survival requires lots of physical activity anyway, this system works well.

Day-to-day life in the industrialized world, on the other hand, has made physical activity optional for many of us. Our lives no longer require and may not even support the level of activity we need for optimal health.

This means we now need to choose to be active even though immediate survival no longer requires it, which is a confusing notion to the emotional brain which still prioritizes rest whenever possible.

The emotional brain rejects most exercise because the only immediate result is effort and inconvenience, along with time taken away from choices that *feel* more readily rewarding, like snacking or seeing what's happening online. There are considerable rewards from exercise, as the questions above reveal, but they happen too far in the future to feel meaningful to the emotional brain.

You know from your cortex that exercise makes life better rather than worse, and does so very reliably. The decision-making power, however, lies in the emotional brain which reacts to exercise as a needless waste of precious energy (unless you've wisely found a way to make it fun, interesting, or challenging, which your emotional brain likes).

When you ask yourself questions like those above, your cortex gives your emotional brain the evidence that it needs in order to *feel* differently about exercise, at least for long enough to get it started on a given day. The cortex basically helps the emotional brain to make its way to a point in the future that is very rewarding to the emotional brain once it gets there, but which it couldn't choose on its own. Here's a quote that sums it up well:

"I'm glad I didn't exercise today," said by no one, ever.[3]

There is one noteworthy exception to all of this, and that is exercising when in poor health. If you are ill or have an injury, exercise only as directed by your doctor. Exercise can often be modified to remain beneficial even though your body is somewhat compromised, but sometimes, you just need to leave the body all of its resources for the work of healing. It's better to get some knowledgeable advice than to either miss out unnecessarily, or conversely, do unintentional harm.

If you have been overweight and out of shape for some time, there is a larger gap in time between the act of exercise and the rewards it brings. You may find that initially, it's unpleasant to move simply because you're stiff, have little muscle strength, and get winded easily. You may essentially need a period of rehab—getting yourself more flexible and acclimated to moving—before you can undertake anything that begins to improve your fitness.

This interim period can be difficult because exercise may well feel worse before it feels better. The key is to lean into the process as much as you safely can, to get the hard part over with as quickly as possible. This means the cortex has to work harder to support an even more reluctant emotional brain in getting started. You might find it helpful to consider the following as they relate to your physical and emotional wellbeing:

- Do you think you'd be better off now if you'd been more physically active over the past year? Do you wish now that you had?

- What is likely to change for you over the next year if you work on getting through this difficult transition so that you can become more physically active? How about five years from now?

- What is likely to change for you over the next year if you don't do this because it feels too hard? How about five years from now?

Each difficult step you take today is one step closer to greater mobility, decreased pain, and more options for enjoying the rest of your life. There is only one way to get those benefits, and that is to start now.

Misdefining Exercise, Part Two

For the majority of human history, exercise was necessarily and seamlessly integrated into daily life, including the work of caring for our families. Now, it's something that needs to be done intentionally rather than occurring naturally in the course of each day. And it has to be fit into a lifestyle where many people feel there's just not enough time for all they need and want to do. With so many competing needs and interests, exercise has lost priority and is now viewed as optional or even self-indulgent, taking time away from the family rather than contributing to it. Many people find the whole idea too guilt-provoking to even consider.

This is a dangerous belief system that must be challenged. Many of us approach health and fitness as if they are primarily about aesthetics but in reality, they deserve the same priority as preventive medical care because they accomplish the same thing: higher quality of life in the present and avoidance of dangerous, expensive, life-stealing medical problems in the future.

We need to stay in good condition to take the best care we can of our families, and to minimize our risk of becoming dependent on them in our older age. We need to lead the way in showing our children the benefits of strong health and the strategies for maintaining it, because no one else will have the influence on their future personal habits that we do. The fact that it improves our own lives along the way just makes it even better.

Adding It All Up

The present-oriented emotional brain predictably misreads modern threats and opportunities. As a result, we find ourselves powerfully drawn to choices which provide but a moment's benefit in exchange for future harm and suffering—suffering which, it must be reiterated, will be endured *by* the emotional brain when the time comes. You've experienced this every time you've overeaten, overspent, lost too many hours to pointless online activity, chosen to date or marry someone who was clearly going to be a bad partner for you, or made any number of other bad choices that felt too compelling at the time to make any other way.

With active effort, you can use your cortex—always in a supportive, caring manner—to help save your emotional brain from itself and come up with strategies that are rewarding in the moment while also setting up a future your emotional brain will enjoy a lot when the time comes.

Questions to yourself, like those mentioned earlier in this chapter, are the key to helping the emotional brain connect the dots and feel more accepting of choices that will work out well in the end. The process is one of bringing lessons from the past and the consequences of the future into sharper present focus for the emotional brain, where it can feel the reality of them and therefore feel more motivated by them. In doing so, you feel a softening of urgency and a greater interest in preserving real happiness and personal integrity. It becomes genuinely easier to act in your own best interests. Not easy, necessarily, but easier.

Any questions you use must be simple and evoke clear, feeling-based memories that will help the emotional brain to shift its focus, one decision at a time. Don't be surprised if you sometimes have to do this multiple times in a single day, because that's actually quite common. The emotional brain seldom retains this kind of learning very well, so you'll find that the clarity you experience one moment won't necessarily help you in the next.

Consider a generic example. Imagine someone has gifted you with one of your favorite treats, a cake from the most renowned bakery in your area. Here's an example of how the internal dialogue might sound:

Emotional brain (EB): "OOOH, CAKE!! Give me a fork and get out of my way!"

Cortex: "I know you think eating a bunch of this right now is going to be great, but it's probably going to turn out badly."

EB: "Shut up; I'll be fine. I love cake! It's my favorite kind, too. I hardly ever get to have this. This is such a special treat, I can't pass it up. We can do healthy stuff some other day."

Cortex: "You can definitely do this if you want to. I can't stop you. But I've been with you every time you've done this before and I don't remember that it ever turned out well. How many times do you remember doing this and being really glad afterward that you did?"

EB: "Well, none, now that you mention it. But geez, it looks and smells so great."

Cortex: "Okay, how many times can you remember doing this and really wishing afterward that you hadn't?"

EB: "Lots. Actually, I think that's happened every time."

Cortex: "Had you expected it to be wonderful all those times, too?"

EB: "Yeah."

Cortex: "How did it actually turn out?"

EB: "I felt bloated and horrible and I hated myself. I don't want that."

Cortex: "This isn't actually a special opportunity either, by the way. The cake happens to be sitting in front of you at the moment, but the bakery makes these every day. There's nothing to be excited about because these are always available."

EB: "Well, that's true."

Cortex: "Would you be willing to go do something else for a little while—a short walk, maybe? That might help you to calm down and get a better idea of what's really going to make you the happiest overall."

EB: "I can do that, but I still might come back and just have cake."

Cortex: "You might, but maybe you'll realize you feel okay about doing something different after all. At least this way, you have a chance to get something better than all the misery you remember from the other times. We can work on a way to have the cake more safely, or maybe we'll figure out that there *is* no way to have it and still be okay in the end. However it turns out, taking some more time to figure it out can't hurt."

EB: "I'm okay with that. I can go walk a little bit, first."

At this point, the emotional brain has loosened up enough to consider some other alternatives. The cortex will actively continue to assist in developing options that the emotional brain can accept, and which will keep the emotional brain the happiest in the end.

So, let's say you walk yourself through this whole process one day, and arrive with great relief and gratitude at a better outcome. Someday not long after, if you see the cake again, here's what's likely to happen:

EB: "OOOH, CAKE!!! Give me a fork and get out of my way!"

And so it goes. The emotional brain and cortex will have the same conversation all over again, as if the previous one had never occurred. The emotional brain can gain genuinely greater clarity for long enough to steer in a safer direction on a per-occasion basis, but due to its limited capabilities, it probably won't retain much from the experience. The lesson will then be largely lost, to be rediscovered all over again the next time, and again the time after that, and so on. You can expect to walk yourself through the facts this way many, many times for the rest of your life. That's perfectly okay because you'll have a far happier life if you do.

It helps to have patience and a sense of humor about this, by the way. Your emotional brain has a limited ability to learn, and it always will. If you can stop telling yourself how this process should be easier or different and just focus on working effectively with the way it actually is, you'll have the most success.

Rest assured, the more you do it, the faster and smoother the process becomes. An internal bit of work such as that described above can easily take place in less than a minute once you've gotten the hang of it. The rewards are well worth it, and it is your emotional brain that will be enjoying them.

Chapter 16
Misuse of the Brain in Decision-Making

You now know that you approach your world with two essentially separate yet intertwined brains, and that the tendencies and strategies of those brains are significantly different. Each is necessary for effective navigation through life, but each has a distinct set of strengths and weaknesses. Some decisions are best suited to the emotional brain and some are best left to the cortex, but most are best served by the coordinated efforts of the two. Life turns out best when you approach each challenge with the part(s) of your brain best equipped for it.

If there is imminent danger where seconds count, for example, it is likely to be the lightning-fast response of your emotional brain that saves the day. If you've ever snatched yourself or a loved one out of harm's way faster than you could form a thought about what was happening, you can credit the emotional brain for making that possible. The cortex's analytical approach at such a time could be so time-consuming as to increase your risk in a situation requiring quick action.

When it comes to something more complicated and conceptual like the management of household finances though, the cortex has to take the lead role. Managing money requires long-term planning, prioritizing, and realistic assessment of resources—all skills that only the cortex has. If this task is left to the emotional brain—something many people actually *do*—it routinely results in mounting debt and financial stress. Financial management is a survival skill specific to the modern world, meaning it presents threats and opportunities the emotional brain cannot understand.

The task of choosing a life partner is a good example of the kind of decision best handled by the cortex and emotional brain together. The emotional brain alone would pick someone based purely on attraction, regardless of how terrible a partner that person might otherwise be. The cortex alone would choose someone trustworthy and reliable, but who might inspire no emotional connectedness at all. In either case, the outcome would probably be a difficult relationship. The odds of success increase considerably when the cortex does the initial screening based on the longer-term merits of potential partners, with the emotional brain then choosing the most attractive of those who make the cut.

Matching Your Brain to the Task

We've previously explored the notion that the modern world presents challenges that are incompatible with the tendencies of the emotional brain. When you use the emotional brain to solve modern problems, you most often get bad results not because there is something wrong with you, but because many modern problems require capabilities that no emotional brain has. Nowhere does this play out more visibly and painfully than it does with issues related to health.

The difficulties start right at the beginning, with how we define the problem. If you hope to solve a problem effectively, you must first identify it accurately. When I ask my audiences what problem caused them to come to my seminar, most people will answer that it's their weight, while just a few might answer that it's their overeating.

"Weight" is an emotional brain answer. The emotional brain focuses on the most obvious source of distress and it seeks a solution targeted very specifically to the problem it has identified. It wants the weight gone—quickly—and will gravitate toward strategies which seem to promise that.

"Overeating" is an answer generated from the cortex. The cortex recognizes that weight is a problem, but that it is secondary to the overeating which caused it. The cortex concludes that if the primary problem of overeating is addressed, the secondary problem of weight will begin to resolve on its own. The cortex will thus choose strategies very different from those favored by the emotional brain.

Since the way a problem is defined dictates the strategies chosen to address it, problem definition also determines the likely success or failure of the effort. This is important to consider since many of us have entrenched and distorted beliefs about weight, food, and eating which keep us stuck misdefining the problem and choosing the same ineffective strategies over and over again. Since we have fewer blind spots in most other areas, it may be easiest to first explore the differing strategies of the emotional brain and cortex as they apply to a problem that is unrelated to food.

Let's say that you've discovered some recent water damage in your basement. The emotional brain and cortex will each notice the same initial signs—wet things, bad smell, perhaps some mold—but from there, the paths quickly diverge.

> The cortex will define the problem as the fact that somehow, water managed to end up where it doesn't belong. The cortex will proceed on the assumption that while immediate cleanup is necessary, it is ultimately most important to figure out what allowed the water to get there in the first place and to fix *that* so there will be no recurrence.
>
> The self-talk may be along the lines of, *I don't like having to deal with this, but at least I can make sure I never have to go through it again.* The basement stays dry for good after the necessary changes have been made, leaving the cortex free to focus itself on other things. The repairs will be casually monitored over time to assure that they're holding up okay.

The process above is, in fact, how most people approach this particular problem. Because we don't have distorted preconceptions when it comes to the issue of a leaky basement, we just get on with the business of fixing it for the long term when we're faced with it. This same dilemma, left only to the discretion of the emotional brain, will be approached in a completely different way:

> The emotional brain will define the problem based on the most obvious and immediately distressing issue—the water itself. The emotional brain's whole focus will be on getting rid of the water and getting the cleanup over with as quickly as possible.
>
> The self-talk might be along the lines of, *It's not fair that I should have to deal with this. I hate it and I don't have time for it. Other people don't have to do it and I don't want to have to do it either.*
>
> Upon completing the cleanup, the emotional brain feels jubilant at having a dry basement once again, and also about being freed from the burden of dealing with the problem. It won't get to enjoy this for very long, however. Since the source of the water was never addressed, more water will inevitably return and the emotional brain will go through the whole cycle all over again, always seeking the fastest path to immediate relief, feeling resentful and burdened each time.

The emotional brain will slowly adjust to living with a chronically damp, musty basement requiring periodic clean-ups, resigning itself to the belief that life just has to be this way. Eventually coming to accept all of this as normal, the emotional brain will actually forget what a consistently dry, comfortable home is like and will no longer aspire to having one.

The emotional brain's approach to a household water problem is ineffective and is not what many people would actually do. It might even sound silly and improbable. Water in this case is a substance that shows up where it is not wanted, which is something you could also say about fat on an overweight person. Faced with the latter problem, how is an emotional brain likely to respond? Since the description above is a good working template for how the emotional brain does things, it will be repeated below, modified only to address the problem of overweight instead of water.

The emotional brain will define the problem based on the most obvious and immediately distressing issue—excess fat. The emotional brain's whole focus will be on getting rid of the fat and getting to a lower weight as quickly as possible.

The self-talk might be along the lines of, *It's not fair that I should have to deal with this. I hate it and I don't have time for it. Other people don't have to do it and I don't want to have to do it either.*

Upon reaching the target weight, the emotional brain feels jubilant at having a healthier and more attractive body, and also about being freed from the burden of dealing with the problem. It won't get to enjoy this for very long, however. Since the source of the excess fat was never addressed, more fat will inevitably return and the emotional brain will go through the whole cycle all over again, always seeking the fastest path to immediate relief, feeling resentful and burdened each time.

The emotional brain will slowly adjust to living with fluctuating health and yo-yo dieting, resigning itself to the belief that life just has to be this way. Eventually coming to accept all of this as normal, the emotional brain will actually forget how good it feels to have a consistently healthy body and will no longer aspire to having one.

This unfortunate process probably sounds very familiar. You can see how ineffective it is when applied to a household water problem, but it is the way most people actually *do* try to deal with the parallel problem of body fat. The take-home message from this is that the emotional brain does not have the skills to properly identify or solve this type of problem. As long as you keep trying to use your brain that way, your efforts will always end up back in the same painful place and you'll be a bit physically and emotionally the worse for wear after each cycle.

If you use the description of the cortex's process from above as applied to the problem of overweight, you get this:

> The cortex will define the problem as the fact that somehow, fat managed to end up where it doesn't belong. The cortex will proceed on the assumption that while reducing weight is necessary, it is ultimately most important to figure out what allowed the fat to get there in the first place and to fix *that* so there will be no recurrence.
>
> The self-talk may be along the lines of, *I don't like having to deal with this, but at least I can make sure I never have to go through it again.* The body gets fitter and healthier for good after the necessary changes have been made, leaving the cortex free to focus itself on other things. The new habits will be casually monitored over time to assure that they're holding up okay.

The approach of the cortex makes much more sense. Better yet, it is also simpler and less time-consuming. Most importantly, it is actually successful. Clearly, the cortex is the part of the brain that must take the lead in matters of health, weight, and self-care practices, but there's one essential qualifier. The strategies of the cortex must be fully acceptable to the emotional brain or they won't be sustainable over time.

Beyond Dieting

The lament shared by most people who have ever tried and failed to achieve lasting weight control is that they know what works, but can't keep it up over the long term. Recalling the overeaters, dieters, and balanced eaters described in Chapter 12, it may now be easier to understand why dieting—healthy or otherwise—generally fails.

Each of us has an emotional brain and a cortex. In any given moment, we can function primarily in emotional mode, cortex mode, or both. We transition fluidly between modes throughout each day as circumstances require, usually with such ease that we are unaware of the process. Overeaters, dieters, and balanced eaters each have a brain mode that they favor most often when it comes to self-care decisions; it is illuminating to see how this relates to the outcomes they tend to achieve.

Overeaters approach their self-care primarily from their emotional brain, resulting in short-sighted decisions that trade momentary pleasure or relief for long-term suffering and reduced quality of life.

When overeaters get sick of this and embark on nutrition-centered diets, they are launching themselves very purposefully into cortex mode. They decide what must be done and doggedly force themselves to do it, enjoying radically improved results for however long they can keep it up. The cortex is running the diet in an attempt to override the emotional brain's need for immediate gratification, but without a strategy for tending to the emotional brain's needs in an alternate way.

This is why nutrition-centered dieters often feel resentful about what they're doing even as it works very well for them—the emotional brain is left wanting and is just waiting for the diet to be over. Eventually, the emotional brain gets tired of waiting and uses its considerable power advantage to end the diet, often with a vengeance. For lack of real emotional brain buy-in up front, the diet was doomed from the start. The cortex never had the power necessary to pull it off independently.

Fad dieting—medically questionable strategies for the purpose of rapid weight-loss—appears to be what happens when the emotional brain is suffering unwanted consequences enough to want relief, but not enough to allow meaningful input from the cortex. The emotional brain is willing do something different for weight loss as long as it gets to see quick results and doesn't have to maintain the project for very long. How long-term health is affected by such diets is of little interest to the emotional brain, locked as it is in the present.

Dieting has a remarkably high failure rate.[1] While this appears to be due to a complex mix of physical and psychological factors, one thing is clear—diets are most often the province of either the cortex or the emotional brain, but rarely both. When it's the cortex, the diet tends to be a nutritious one which will nonetheless be rejected by the emotional brain as too burdensome and/or unrewarding to maintain. When the emotional brain is in charge, the diet is likely to involve unhealthy or even dangerous strategies that are geared only toward fast results and a short overall project time.

Balanced eaters stand in stark contrast to all this internal friction and frustration by using both the cortex and the emotional brain in a coordinated way most of the time. Their goal is certainly to enjoy momentary pleasures, but only to the extent that there are no unwanted longer-term consequences as a result. This means that they aim to eat in a way that is very enjoyable, but which stops short of incurring costs like guilt, shame, physical discomfort, unwanted weight, and compromised health.

Balanced eaters evaluate potential pleasures—food and otherwise—based on two tests. The first test, involving the emotional brain, is to consider how enjoyable a given choice may be in the moment. The second test, reflecting cortex involvement, is to consider whether the choice adds to or detracts from the *life* you most want for yourself.

Consider a common pattern described by many overeaters: having pizza or other take-out food several times every week. This passes the first test handily, which is why people keep doing it, but the results of the second test are terrible. I have yet to speak with anyone who truly enjoys and prefers the conditions they live with when they routinely make choices of this kind. When balanced eaters want something like pizza, they make sure that they have it enough to enjoy the experience, but not enough for it to interfere with the life that they desire.

Choices made with *both* tests in mind result in day-to-day living that takes good care of the emotional brain in both the present and the future. Such choices also happen to result in superior support of the body as well. Because the emotional brain is consistently satisfied, there is no slow building of fatigue or resentment. There is no falling off the wagon because there *is* no wagon, just a way of living that is relaxed and satisfying day after day.

It is easier, more enjoyable, and more beneficial to adopt the coordinated-brain process of balanced eaters, but there is an important factor preventing most of us from doing it. When the emotional brain gets triggered enough to start to take over, it is difficult or impossible to put oneself in cortex mode due to the survival wiring that gives primacy to the emotional brain.

We've adapted to possess the stubborn, unshakeable determination it takes to succeed at getting enough food to survive in an environment of scarcity, physical hardship, and life-threatening hazards. That determination remains with us despite the fact that our circumstances have changed considerably—we remain powerfully driven to maximize food opportunities even though this is no longer the best survival strategy.

The result is an involuntary and demoralizing loss of control whenever the emotional brain is exposed to triggering situations, a situation that overeaters experience quite frequently. Balanced eaters simply sidestep this problem by living in a manner that minimizes such triggering, allowing them to feel generally in control as they maintain calm, enjoyable lives.

Balanced eaters in the modern world have the same emotional brain that everyone else has. Most of them would become overeaters if they had to live in chronically triggering conditions, so they make sure they live in more favorable conditions.

They don't necessarily have stronger innate tendencies toward healthier practices, but they definitely have a more intentional approach to how they live. They plan and set up their lives very purposefully—using the cortex—in ways that make it easier to maintain healthy patterns, and that also keep their emotional brains both satisfied and safe. A satisfied and safe emotional brain stays calm enough to keep the cortex in the loop, allowing for the quality decision-making that keeps the good times rolling.

Chapter 17
Deep Change Takes Time

As noted in Chapter 9, the emotional brain develops strong biases which it holds onto rather stubbornly once they've formed. Anyone in recovery from addiction will tell you that such biases can be changed, but that it's not easy and it takes a lot of focus over a long time to achieve. This in itself is greatly frustrating to the emotional brain, which wants what it wants *now*, including recovery once that has become the objective.

Most of the overeaters with whom I've worked have shared a quiet hope that I could give them something to do—however arduous—that would be time-limited and would permanently end their drive to overeat. They might seriously consider a "therapy" of walking on hot coals every day for a month, for example, if doing so could guarantee effortlessly controlled eating for the rest of their lives.

Ironically, the same people who would bring genuine, raw determination to such an ordeal usually can't bear the thought of the far simpler lifestyle changes that reliably work, but which must be maintained on an ongoing basis. This is because the emotional brain focuses on the present—which does not favor long-term projects—and tends to hold onto familiar patterns rather than adopting new ones.

There are two general ways in which you might get your emotional brain to change a bias that is proving disruptive to the life you'd like to have: a fast way and a slow way. In keeping with the emotional brain's fondness for things that are fast, we'll look at that one first.

The Fast Track
The fast path to emotional change involves having a life experience of such intensity that established biases are shattered, opening the way for something new. A positive example of this is spiritual enlightenment—a startling moment of clarity after which the world never again looks the same. These experiences are wonderful, but few people ever have them.

The negative version of the moment-of-change experience is some form of trauma. In the world of eating issues, that trauma is usually a dramatic, life-threatening health crisis like a heart attack. You can hear from your doctor about your diabetes for years on end and never have it approach the impression made by the terror of one heart attack, ambulance ride, and stay in your local ICU.

Some people ignore their health for decades until this particular crisis arrives, after which they clean out the pantry and the fridge, start hitting the gym, and lose a hundred pounds in the first year based entirely on lifestyle change. Sadly, however, many others experience exactly the same crisis but instead, stop at their local drive-through for burgers practically on their way home from the hospital.

Slow and Steady Wins the Race

The fast path to emotional change, whether spiritually uplifting or traumatically devastating, is simply too unreliable to be a viable solution to the problem of overeating. That leaves the more mundane slow path that is a long time in the making. While the fast path is one dramatic event after which everything feels forever different, the slow path is the accumulation over time of many more ordinary events and experiences that, by way of sheer repetition, gradually shift the biases of the emotional brain.

This process is implied in the old saying, "Fake it 'til you make it," a concept which is well respected among those who deal with addiction and recovery. It means that if you want recovery from an addiction, you will have to spend time doing the things that recovering people do even though, in your heart, you're not there yet.

The idea is that if you act like a recovering person for long enough—enjoying the benefits of those better decisions along the way even though your heart isn't in it—you'll eventually discover that somewhere along the way you've actually *become* a recovering person, and that it was worth the effort. In other words, go through the motions for long enough and the feelings will follow.

You may now be thinking about your past experiences with some frustration: *But what about all those times I went on a diet? What about all those times I ate better food, had smaller portions, exercised more, and took better care of myself? Sometimes I did it for months! How come none of that ever stuck?*

There is an oft-repeated adage that if you do something consistently for 30 days, it will become a habit; the implication is that it will become automatic for you once you've made it through the first month. This idea has done a lot of damage by creating the expectation that if you can just hang on by your fingernails to some new behavior for a limited amount of time, you'll lose your urges to the contrary.

When that doesn't happen as expected, many people give up and quit altogether. The 30-day timeframe may be effective for something simple like learning to leave your car keys in the same place every day or remembering where everything is after you've reorganized your closets, but it barely scratches the surface for making real shifts in the emotional brain.

Change in the emotional brain's biases, when it happens at all, happens across a span of months or years, not days or weeks. This means you can go through the motions of better health practices for a long time before you begin to feel personally motivated toward those practices other than as a means to an end for losing weight or averting some medical disaster. You get verifiable benefits all along the way, of course, like feeling better, more energy, weight loss, and improvement of chronic medical conditions. As worthwhile as those benefits are, they lack the intensity and immediacy that would get the emotional brain's interest enough to really *want* to pursue them.

Consider a thought experiment in which you give your emotional brain a choice between lower blood pressure and a doughnut (or whatever other food it is that gets you going). Your emotional brain will always react more strongly to the doughnut, simply because the doughnut has intense sensory appeal and can be readily obtained, two characteristics that carry enormous weight with the emotional brain.

By comparison, the reward of lower blood pressure generates less emotional excitement and worse, comes only after a substantial delay. That, in a nutshell, is why it can feel so hard to stay the course even when you can see very good reasons for doing so.

It is in maintaining your new practices for a long time, continually accruing and benefiting from the more subtle rewards, that the emotional brain eventually starts to see the connection. Rather than one huge lesson that changes everything in an instant, it is thousands of tiny lessons over time that eventually make an impression.

For example, the emotional brain expects to dislike exercise but is pleasantly surprised to feel good—at least after the fact—about doing it. It expects to get the best reward from eating as much as possible, but discovers that it's a tremendous relief to be able to stop eating before becoming uncomfortably bloated. Lessons like these quietly accumulate over months and years until eventually, the emotional brain starts to get the point. When that happens, you begin to *want* the choices that really make life better, rather than merely wishing you wanted them.

Until this internal shift occurs, you are tasked with practicing the mini-lessons the many times it will take for your emotional brain finally to make the connection, all while dealing with its resistance along the way. Given how powerful the emotional brain is, this might sound like an impossible task. In fact, learning how to work more effectively with your emotional brain is much easier than the doomed task of trying to overcome it.

There is considerable reason for cheer in this, because it means that compared to what you've probably been doing up to this point, you can labor less while getting better results for your efforts. That's an outcome that any emotional brain will welcome, so rest assured this is not just an uphill battle that never pays off until you're too tired to care anymore.

Chapter 18
The Body of Your Dreams vs.
the Body in Your Mirror

Most overeaters are overweight; it is their weight and its consequences that motivate most to consider change. I address the issue of weight here with some reluctance because the point of this book is the management of eating, not weight. They are related, of course, but they are *not* the same thing.

I am touching on the topic of weight loss primarily because I know it is the most likely reason you started reading this book. If you happen to be obese, there are some important facts about weight loss and weight management that must be acknowledged so that you know what to expect and are empowered to achieve the best results you can.

Many overweight people come to see their weight as the source of most that is wrong in their lives, believing that losing it will make everything right again. Many hope that once the weight is gone, their body will be restored to what it would be had there been no period of overweight in the first place. For those who are obese, this won't be entirely true.

While the self-repair capabilities of the human body are incredible, it does have limits. It can recover completely from many insults, provided those insults do not occur repetitively over a long enough period of time. There are many things we do to our bodies though, that will eventually create lasting physical change even after we've stopped the behavior in question, like the carpal tunnel syndrome we get from too much time spent at a keyboard or the chronic respiratory problems we may live with long after we quit smoking.

It happens that the same is true of being overweight. We are all capable of gaining some amount of weight, carrying it for some period of time, and still being capable of a full physical recovery once we've shed the excess pounds. We each have a point though—highly variable among individuals—after which we've carried too much weight or carried it for too long to be able to go all the way back to our physical and metabolic baseline once we've lost it.

Weight loss will result in remarkable benefits no matter when you do it, but the results that are possible for you may be different from what you hope for if you've carried your extra weight for many years. The solution is to go in with realistic expectations in the first place so you can stay focused on making the most of what is possible for you.

Aesthetic Issues in Significant Weight Loss

There are numerous health-related reasons to reduce excess weight, but most people start thinking about it mainly because they want to look better. Losing a *lot* of weight can produce a mixed bag of results— it improves your overall health and certain aspects of your appearance, yet can actually create some new appearance problems along the way.

Skin is amazing in its ability to stretch and accommodate any amount of weight you can gain. What it can't always do is regain its shape and tone after the excess weight has been shed, depending on several variables:

- The more your skin has been stretched and the longer it has stayed that way, the greater your likelihood of excess skin issues when you lose weight.

- The more weight you lose, the more skin will be left essentially emptied of the excess fat it once held.

- The faster you lose weight, the harder it is for the skin to keep up in terms of adjusting to your changing shape.

- Everyone's skin loses elasticity as we age, so the older you are when you lose weight, the greater the chance that your skin won't keep up.

- Your overall health and genetic heritage also affect your body's ability to recover once you've gotten it to a healthier weight.

If these variables don't align enough in your favor, you may be left with flaps and folds of excess skin after weight loss, particularly in the abdominal area, upper arms, and thighs. In addition to the aesthetic disadvantages, excess skin is harder to keep clean and can be the site of chafing and skin infections.

Some people deal with these issues by undergoing expensive, painful surgery for skin reduction. Others just take extra care with personal hygiene, tuck the folds into the flattering clothing they can now wear, and get on with their greatly improved lives, grateful for the world of possibilities that has opened to them. Some, unfortunately, become so discouraged by what they see that they abandon their efforts altogether.

No one wants to end up dealing with excess skin and perhaps you won't have to, but it may be a price you pay in exchange for the weight loss that grants you improved health and more ability to pursue the activities in life that you enjoy the most. If you go into the process with realistic expectations, you will be able to make the most of your results, whatever they are.

You've Been Getting Older, You Know

Most people who have a significant amount of weight to lose have carried it for some time. Many in their middle and older years undergo weight loss with the unconscious expectation that they will get back something approaching the build they had the last time they were at their current target weight. This is an unrealistic expectation because it fails to take into account the fact that if you've carried excess weight for years, you are now years older than you used to be.

You can always get back a much better body than you've been used to recently and weight loss will slow your future rate of physical aging, but it can't roll back the effects of aging that has already taken place.

You won't get back quite the same shape, because body mass tends to shift downward over time. There will be some areas that you can no longer tighten up no matter what you do now, other than surgery. That's because this is the body you'd have had by now anyway, and not because weight loss has somehow betrayed you.

It's only after some weight is out of the way that you can see how you're actually built at this stage in your life. Again, realistic expectations at the outset will keep you moving forward, making the most of what is possible for you.

Ongoing Maintenance Challenges

Research confirms what many people have long believed—if you've lost a lot of weight, keeping it off seems harder than it should be.[1] If you are obese for an extended period of time, your body may undergo internal changes that affect you for the rest of your life even after you've lost much of the extra weight.

For example, if you spend years at 300 pounds and then lose 100 of them, you might end up metabolically different from an otherwise identical person who weighed 200 pounds all along. If this is the case, your body will have become far more efficient in energy management,[2] needing as much as 20-25% fewer calories per day[3] to maintain the same weight as that person of the same size who was never obese. That's several hundred calories per day of less-food/more-exercise you'll have to maintain just to break even once you've gotten down to the weight you wish to keep.

Unfortunately, the simple fact of getting older works against you as well. Our caloric needs decrease across our lifespan for many reasons, not least being the fact that we all tend to lose some muscle mass and develop more fat deposits as we age.

Muscle is more metabolically active (it needs more energy) than fat, so losing muscle means the body needs less energy overall—you gradually need fewer calories in a day to keep breaking even as you age.[4,5] Decreasing muscle mass also means decreasing ability to maintain activity of the intensity that may have typified your younger years, thus lowering your daily caloric needs even further.

As much as we in the developed world may bemoan our inability to get away with eating like we used to, it's actually a tremendous survival advantage in the wild. When you're getting older, slower, less powerful, and don't bounce back from setbacks as well as you used to, it's a good thing to require less food. It means that you don't have to work as hard or take as many risks in order to stay adequately fed.

Decreasing energy needs and increasing energy storage are the perfect adaptation for aging successfully ... in the wild. For those of us who have learned to prize eating more for emotional rewards than for physical benefits though, not so much.

Why It's Still Best to Lose Whatever Weight You Can

Perhaps you're now thinking that while being overweight is a trying way to live, what you're left with after losing weight doesn't sound much better. Why would anyone bother going through the trouble of change if it's just trading one set of problems for another? Maybe it looks like your best shot at a happy life now is to just live with what you have and skip what seems like pointless and endless effort.

That's probably not true, and here's why.

Being overweight is hard. If you are overweight, you will live with more fatigue, more pain, and spend your life at greater risk for depression.[6] You will be more vulnerable to opportunistic infections and chronic diseases. You will have fewer options for engaging in your life and enjoying time with your loved ones.

If you're obese, it takes as little as a 5-10% reduction in body weight[7] to improve your medical status and your quality of life. If you can't or don't care to shed all of your excess pounds, losing *some* of them will still give you more choices, more freedom, and more ways to enjoy life than you've had access to for years.

No matter what weight you're starting from, you have the power to make your life better and more worthwhile with every lost pound—every one of them matters. If you start out 100 pounds overweight and level off after losing 25, for example, you will still have dramatically improved your quality of life and the outlook for your future.

The more of the excess you can lose, the better,[8] but losing anything at all will make a difference that you can feel and enjoy, *provided you are willing to accept it.*

Remember the hazard of all-or-nothing thinking which whispers cruel and misleading things like, *Sure, you've lost 25 pounds but look how far there still is to go. Who are you kidding? What's the point? You'll never beat this, so you might as well at least enjoy yourself.* Self-talk like that invites you to settle into a life of needless limitation, illness, and burden. Even if you can't get the body you really want, you can always get one that serves you better, keeps you happier, and allows you a much better life than the one you will have if you give up.

Chapter 19
Maintaining Motivation

Motivation is the reason we want to do something, and the level of interest we feel in following through. Positive motivation can be a powerful mix of high-energy feelings like inspiration, focus, determination, and hope. When you feel motivated, anything seems possible.

If only you could feel that way more of the time.

Common Motivators That Often Don't Seem to Work

Inconsistent motivation is the life story of most overeaters, to their great dismay. It seems that all have at one time or another—usually, many times—felt enthusiastically locked onto their goals for personal change, only to have their interest fade over time or get displaced by other demands in life.

The vast majority of these people share a common source of motivation: weight loss. This shows you that weight loss as a primary objective is simply ineffective at motivating most people over the long term. If focusing on weight was an adequate motivator, we would have no obesity problem. Few people would ever gain weight more than once, because the problem would be self-correcting.

Concern about weight *feels* like a powerful motivator. In that moment when you decide you just can't stand it anymore and really have to make some changes, you have emotional intensity that could fuel almost any effort. With that level of focus, it doesn't matter whether it's easy or convenient because you're determined to make it work.

The problem is that the intensity isn't sustainable; at some point, it fades. When that happens, it doesn't matter how well you have set yourself up to succeed. You can have the best fitness equipment, plenty of money to buy quality food, and lots of time to do whatever is necessary but without motivation, nothing will happen. This is why you may have fitness equipment rusting in your basement and vegetables rotting in your refrigerator. Many people hope the mere physical presence of such things will inspire motivation or at least spur action through guilt, but the reality is that it rarely works.

To be clear, concern about weight alone *can* be sufficient motivation for some people. The problem is that the group for whom this reliably works is so small. The rest of us need motivation with stronger staying power.

Many people try to focus on achieving better health. Others can't find any personal goal that sticks well enough, so they try to focus on setting a better example for their children.

As with focusing on weight, there are some people for whom these motivators work quite well. Those who are motivated by concern for their health and/or that of their children tend more often to achieve lasting results than do those who are driven primarily by the number on the bathroom scale. Unfortunately though, they still experience a high failure rate. Many ultimately lose track of their goals and resume their old habits, even with motivators as compelling as these.

This might make it seem like few people care much about their own health or about that of their children, but that makes no sense—of course they care. Once again, we may find a way to understand this by looking at the functioning of the brain.

Strong Motivation Comes from the Emotional Brain

Ironically, the problem shared by the motivators described above may be that they all make such good sense. "Good sense" implies heavy cortex involvement, meaning the cortex has looked at all the available information, considered long-term probable outcomes, and has concluded that behaviors that foster good health in ourselves and our kids are the way to go. Brilliant. So why are the vast majority of people failing to follow through?

Part of the problem is that the emotional brain is most strongly influenced by whatever seems most compelling in the moment.

We know in our cortex that quality food makes us feel better and will support a better life, but that dessert on the table looks so good *right now*. We know we need to instill healthy habits in our kids for their long-term welfare, but treats and sodas make them so happy *right now*, and we enjoy seeing them happy. Those foods may also get the kids to quit bugging us *right now*, which is important when we're stressed and tired. We know we need to take more time to stock up on and prepare quality food, but the drive-through is so much easier *right now*. We know it would be a good idea to get some exercise but it feels more important to get to other items on the to-do list *right now*. And so it goes with sensible choices getting overruled, one after another, in favor of what is easiest or most rewarding in the moment.

The emotional brain seeks reward now—it's not motivated by grand plans that pay off in the distant future. This is why it often pulls harder toward a plate of cookies than it does toward the diabetes you hope to avoid or the long-term habits you're hoping to instill in your kids.

It isn't that your goals are unimportant; it's simply that they often fail to generate enough immediate reward to compete with whatever else has gotten your emotional brain's attention.

We try to compensate for this by adding momentum to the goal in other ways. New Year's resolutions—famous for their high failure rate—are a perfect example of trying to drum up some excitement in the emotional brain even though it is not truly on board with the idea. It's a somewhat desperate attempt to get a boost from the new-year/fresh-start concept, but you don't hear of many long-term success stories that launched on the first of January.

If that doesn't work, we may try entering a weight loss contest or other health challenge at work, hoping to catch a boost from feeling competitive or the chance at tangible rewards like money or a favored parking space.

It isn't that these programs never work, but that the results are so often transitory in nature. For example, a personal friend of mine famously won his workplace weight loss challenge several years in a row. No, he wasn't fitter and healthier from one year to the next; he simply regained all the weight each year. The contest never resulted in any lasting behavioral change. Worse, it reliably triggered an annual bout of unhealthy weight loss tactics that also happened to get him some extra cash.

Sometimes we try to increase the emotional brain's interest by giving it some company; we do this when we buddy up with a friend to pursue health-related goals together. Sometimes we engage that friend as a personal probation officer, hoping that if we have someone to whom we feel accountable, we'll do more of the right thing due to social pressure even if we still feel otherwise unenthused about the project.

We try strategies like these in the hope that if we can just go through the motions long enough, the new patterns will begin to stick and we won't have to keep trying so hard. As explained in Chapter 17, there is some logic to this; the problem is that we dramatically underestimate how long it will take, and also fail to keep the emotional brain adequately rewarded in the interim. Days or weeks into the process—months if we're doing better than most people—we tire from the effort and abandon it for what we really want, which is the behavior we were trying to talk ourselves into changing.

That's the problem. We fail when we try to ignore what we really want. What we really want generally prevails in the end, for better or worse, so that's the only place the battle can ever truly be won.

Your emotional brain is capable of powerful motivation. You feel it every time you give in to an irresistible food urge because in that moment, you are motivated toward the comfort and relief you expect from the immediate sensory pleasure of the food. Imagine what you could accomplish if you could channel that motivation more constructively.

Your first step in that direction is to identify the personal goals that your cortex knows will support the kind of life you'd really rather have. Next, you'll need to develop ways to keep your emotional brain supported and satisfied every step along the way.

Identifying Goals That Matter to *You*
Your longer-term goals will seldom have the immediate motivating power required by your emotional brain, but it's still important to frame them in the most emotionally relevant terms that you can. As mentioned earlier, most people focus on weight, yet we know that most don't remain motivated by that over time. If the focus on weight is not working anyway, there's no risk in trying something different.

Focus more than you have in the past on *why* you want to control your weight. How do you imagine or hope your life will be different when you do? What new sources of enjoyment and opportunity will become available? What problems will be reduced or eliminated? What physical and emotional pains might you expect to alleviate and what might your life be like with fewer of them?

The answers to questions like these will show you your real goals, so take the time to consider them and flesh them out in detail that makes them real to you on an emotional level. If you can't *feel* the importance of the goal it will lack the power you need it to have, regardless of how sensible it may be. You need to identify goals that you truly care about and that you're likely to keep caring about for years to come even as life throws distractions at you along the way.

Most people have these deeper reasons that prompt them to take on weight control in the first place. The problem starts when they begin focusing on the weight itself more than on the personal goals that started the process; that's when interest weakens and the process falls apart. Better general health is the most socially repeated reason for changing personal habits, yet is probably the reason of least interest to the emotional brain. You're better off identifying more specific goals that are highly personalized to the life you want. Here are some that have been meaningful for people I have known:

- The ability to buy more attractive clothing.
- The ability to buy clothing in mainstream stores.
- The ability to play on the floor with children or grandchildren.
- Preventing diabetes and other looming medical threats.
- Reducing the need for medications.
- Preserving mobility.
- Reducing pain.
- Maintaining physical independence in older age.
- The ability to feel in control.
- Preventing or minimizing depression.
- The physical ability to engage in activities of personal interest by being able to fit in seats in public venues and having the strength and stamina required for desired sports or hobbies.

It's important for any goal you select to have emotional impact for you. *You must then keep your primary focus on that goal and your progress toward it, rather than on your weight.*

For example, if your goal is to be able to play on the floor with kids, you'll want to focus on eating foods that provide lasting energy to keep you going, and which have low inflammatory qualities in order to reduce your pain. You'll also need to move around a lot more in general to maximize your flexibility and strength. As it happens, those choices also support good health and are likely to result in the loss of a few of the excess pounds you may be carrying.

If you keep your focus on doing what it takes to move toward what you really want, you'll naturally make choices that have a positive impact on your health. Pursue what you want with determination and you basically get better health for free. This is a wonderful win-win for your emotional brain.

Your self-assessment questions should always be, *Am I getting closer to being able to do what I want? If not, what do I need to change so I can make more progress?* rather than, *What's happening with my weight?* Focusing on what you want is more effective and also feels a lot better.

Any goal has the potential to be either useful or not, depending on the individual. If it doesn't inspire you to think about having better health but you *can* get excited about wearing cuter clothes, for example, then by all means, do it for the clothes! All that matters is that you find something you *want* to grab onto and that is likely to hold your interest over time. Ideally, it's something you want enough to fight for it a bit when you have to, because you don't want it taken away from you.

As long as your goal gives you energy for change and creates no harm, you're good to go. If you can't identify a single goal that has the emotional impact you need to get in gear, it may be possible to tap sufficient motivational energy from several lesser goals that together, provide enough to get the job done.

For example, it may not motivate you enough when you think of being able to fly commercially without a seatbelt extender, or being able to breathe freely even when you have to bend over for something, or being able to reach your feet so that you can take better care of them, but maybe those three things together (or others like them) will generate enough combined reward to get you mobilized.

Anything can work. It's just a question of figuring out what can work for *you*. It may take some determined self-assessment to figure out what will work best for you, but it is time and effort well invested.

Don't be discouraged when your interest wanes sometimes anyway, despite your having identified a deeply compelling personal reason to make some changes. In fact, you can expect it. The most wisely chosen and personally relevant goals will still sometimes fail to provide the ongoing and immediate reward that your emotional brain needs on a day-to-day basis.

Not to worry—you can still keep your emotional brain well cared for every step of the way, and it's essential that you do so. You need consistent engagement of your cortex in order to live successfully in the modern world, and you'll only have that if the emotional brain remains content enough to release control over decision-making. Reliable care of the emotional brain's needs is critical to long-term success, so you'll find a great deal of information devoted to the matter in Part Four.

Chapter 20
Daring to be Different

In Part One, we examined the eating and activity patterns now practiced by the majority of people around us, which likely includes most if not all of your closest family members and dearest friends. We are all members of various relational groups (family, coworkers, neighbors, friends, fellow congregants, etc.), and each of those groups have certain practices that are part of the group's unique identity. Such practices express an underlying theme of "This is how we do things; this is who we are," and many of those practices involve food.

Groups often exert subtle or even open pressure on their members to maintain the status quo, reinforcing the shared practices that strengthen group unity. As such, when you decide to change your eating habits and become more physically active, it can feel like you're breaking ranks even though your feelings for everyone remain the same. Any changes you make will be felt in some way by everyone who is close to you, and they will each have a reaction of some kind.

The best response you can hope for is active support of your efforts. Some friends and family might even come along for the ride and consider some changes themselves. This makes for a happier and easier experience when it works out this way, but is actually not the majority experience.

The next most favorable level of response you might get from others is that while they don't embrace your changes, they also don't interfere in any way. They may look at you as something of an oddity, but they leave you in peace to pursue your strange ideas and they still love you nonetheless. It might feel mildly disappointing if that's the response you get, but at least you can feel comfortable in your relationships and get on with what you need to do. Open support from others is nice when you can get it, but it's not essential.

It gets trickier as you continue along the spectrum of possible responses from others, because what you're left with is active interference with your efforts, whether it's done with misguided good intentions or in an attempt at outright sabotage. It is far beyond the scope of this book to debate how you resolve the dilemma of a relationship with someone whose actions would have you remaining stuck in a way of life that has caused you emotional and physical misery. Many have reached this particular fork in the road and have abandoned their efforts at change rather than risking disturbance in important relationships. That is one of your options and if you choose it, I hope you do so in peace.

If you choose to proceed with changing how you live even though it unsettles the patterns you've previously shared with those around you, the information that follows will help you to prepare for the challenges that may come.

Understanding Social Pressure to Keep Overeating

"Oh come on, it's just a little piece—have some."

"It's a special occasion—loosen up and enjoy yourself."

"Try this. No, seriously, *try* it!"

"Are you *sure* you've had enough?"

You are likely to experience pressure like this from any number of people as you experiment with different choices and patterns in how you eat. It may come from family members who express love through food or who want company in shared overindulgence. Maybe it's the coworker who keeps bringing snacks into the office for everyone. Perhaps you have a neighbor who really likes to bake, and then gives the goodies to nearby friends so she won't have overly tempting foods in her own home.

If you're trying to achieve better control with food, chances are that you'll regularly encounter people who seem to be working actively to make you fail.

This is more understandable when you remember that our social norms around food have their origins in times of food scarcity and hunger, and that those are the conditions for which we remain wired today. For most of human history, it has made perfect sense to fret about your loved ones not getting enough, to give food at every opportunity, and to elevate food to a role of primary personal and social importance.

Our environment has changed but our social norms haven't. The end result is that when someone tries to adopt strategies that are a better fit for our current circumstances, they often experience pushback from the people with whom they live, work, and play.

The present-day motivations that keep food pressure in place are wide-ranging, but mostly benign. Food may be insistently offered out of a sense of duty, fearing that to do less is to fail loved ones. Some people greatly enjoy giving food, and therefore give a *lot* because they find it so satisfying to do so. Shared food is an important element of family bonding, prompting some to try to get everyone to eat the same way regardless of individual need and preference.

On the darker side, some people *do* push food on others in overtly negative ways, often as the expression of a relational power struggle. In more extreme cases, the food pusher may unconsciously be using food specifically to make you fail. Note the sentiment that has been expressed on countless posters and gag gifts: "Dear Lord, if you can't make me thin, then please make all my friends fat."

Misery does indeed love company. If one member of a relational group attempts change and fails, then others may feel relieved of the obligation to try, in addition to finding comfort in the reaffirmation of the group's historic practices. From the standpoint of group cohesion, order has been restored.

"You've lost too much weight. You should eat more."

Your family and friends have known you to look and behave a certain way for a long time and may find it unsettling when you change, even when it's in ways that are to your benefit. You're not only engaging in practices that run counter to "what we do" as a family or other group, you're becoming different from what they're used to. As a result, you may hear concerns about weight loss even though your weight has not fallen to an unhealthy level.

It is useful at this point to remember that until just the last few decades, dramatic changes in appearance due to weight loss have usually been a marker of serious illness or other misfortune. Indeed, many loved ones react to these kinds of appearance changes with a nagging concern that something is wrong. They may worry even as you continue to remain overweight at a level that compromises your health. They may tell you that you look unhealthy.

Some people lose weight from the top down, which can further complicate how friends and family react to the changes in their appearance. They lose weight in their faces first and then primarily in their upper bodies, sometimes while maintaining substantial fat storage from the waist down. You can begin to look somewhat drawn in the face—which is what people notice the most about you—while remaining overweight overall.

It is certainly true that people sometimes *do* resort to questionable methods of weight loss, losing too much weight in too short a time, stressing their bodies terribly in the process, ultimately looking less healthy because that is actually true. Concerned loved ones in these cases are rightfully alarmed.

But what about when you lose a reasonable amount of weight in healthy ways, yet your loved ones still respond with concern because they weren't prepared for how different you might look? Or what if your loved ones are objecting because you are now adopting healthier habits than they have, and they are unconsciously working to persuade you back into compliance with the norms of the group?

If that kind of pressure ever starts to make you question the quality of your choices, you can clear it up easily with a routine medical exam and conversation with your doctor.[1] It is always a good idea to have a reputable physician aware of your status and your self-care patterns in any event, especially if you are getting into middle and older age.

Your loved ones may back down once they've heard that your strategies have been validated by a medical professional, or they may not. At the very least, you'll have the reassurance you need so that you can keep your focus on the goals that matter to you.

Communicating About Change

There are conversations you can try having with some of the people in your life that might help them to better understand what you need on your journey, should they wish to support you more effectively. It is entirely possible that those with whom you speak will thoughtfully take in what you say, pledge to experiment with some changes, and then unconsciously keep doing exactly what they've always done. Overeating is not the only behavior for which there are neural superhighways, after all.

If the people close to you are truly open to trying some new things, it's a good idea to acknowledge how easy it will be for them accidentally to fall back into old habits at times. It's helpful to secure their agreement up front that it's okay for you to point out such slips kindly if they happen. The following topics may give you some ideas to consider as you decide what you'd like to discuss.

It's Easier When Others Don't Prompt Us to Eat

In general, overeaters do best when left to decide for themselves what food, and how much of it, ends up in their world and on their plates. Ideally, this means that others do not offer food, e.g., "I'm getting some ice cream—would you like some?" They don't encourage you to take larger portions, suggest that you take seconds, or prompt you in any other way toward food. There is no need for anyone ever to do those things, because you are quite capable of assessing your food needs and taking care of them yourself. You will do so more easily without others pushing you in that direction.

Most overeaters experience some degree of inner torment when others invite or encourage them to eat. They really want to eat, but they often wish they didn't want to; they fight with themselves inside and usually lose, feeling defeated with food once again as a result.

I have long observed that as much as people agonize over their own internal struggles of this type, they fail to realize that they do *the very same thing* to others whom they might encourage, invite, or pressure to eat. It is likely that you are surrounded by people who, though they struggle with it themselves, are also doing it to you.

Offering food is usually meant as a sign of caring, but for the overeater trying to make some changes, *not* offering is actually the more caring thing to do. Explaining this can be helpful.

It isn't that we must pretend food doesn't exist or vow never to mention it at all. For example, it is quite sufficient at a social gathering to let people know at the beginning of the event where all the food is located (preferably slightly out of the way so people can get away from it if they want to), and to invite them to help themselves as they wish. This way, generosity and nurturing can be offered in ways that help the overeater to stay calm and happy with food, rather than tortured.

The Thorny Issue of Gifted Food

Gifts of food present another variation of the same challenge. Gifting someone with treat food—unless they have told you they would like to receive it—risks putting them into that awful internal conflict which will probably end badly.

The internal battle is actually worse with food gifts, because in addition to struggling with temptation, the recipient is also worrying about the feelings of the gift-giver. If that has been your experience, it might be beneficial to make some requests to family and friends about avoiding such gifts, or at least keeping the size limited.

It is also very thoughtful to consider this issue when you are choosing gifts for others, and perhaps to have conversations with them about what they would really enjoy the most.

Food is often given not so much as a gift as a way to move excess from one person's life into that of another. Two common examples are the host who insists (over guests' objections) that leftovers be taken home, and the coworker who brings in leftovers or unwanted treat food from home "because otherwise, we'll just eat it." The intention is to keep food from being wasted, harkening back to the days when food was a precious resource in finite supply. Since we now live in conditions of harmful abundance, the essential message of such an act is, *This would be a problem for me so, here—you deal with it.*

Such a negative message is surely not what people consciously have in mind when they do such things, but it is the reality of the result; wherever the food lands, it is likely to cause some struggle where there would otherwise have been none. If we can have more conversations with the people around us about this, perhaps we can do less unintentional harm to one another. The key, by the way, is to buy, make, and otherwise obtain less food to start with so there won't be an excess to try to pass around.

Food is Less Tempting When It's Out of Sight

Food storage practices—or lack thereof—are an issue in many homes and workplaces. Sometimes food gets left out in plain sight when it might just as easily be stored away from view. The sight of food is triggering for most people, and food left sitting out invites a great deal of eating that was neither planned nor wanted.

If there are people in your orbit who leave food out unnecessarily— on countertops or coffee tables, for example—they may make more of an effort to keep it out of sight if you help them understand that it is difficult for you. Of course, be sure that you don't inflict this challenge on anyone else, either.

Adding Variety to Time Shared with Others

As detailed in Chapter 2, the way most people spend time together has come to be dominated by food, to the detriment of most of us. Since it is likely that you and your loved ones have fallen into this same pattern without really planning to, it could be interesting to talk about more creative ways to share the time. You'd still eat together, of course, because that's enjoyable and people do need to eat at some point, but what if you had other plans that were the main reason for getting together?

What might it be like if you sometimes planned a walk, a hike, attending an event, volunteering together, playing games, going to a movie or show, or working on a home project together, then sharing a simple meal afterwards while you traded stories about the day?

Sharing food reinforces bonds between members of a relational group, but it is sharing life experiences that gives those bonds strength and depth. There are many great memories to be made, but few of them will happen if all you ever do together is eat.

Chapter 21
Putting It All Together

Every psychological hurdle described in Part Three is here not because I've seen so many people affected by each one, but because I've seen so many people affected by *most or all of them at the same time*. When you go through life this way without awareness or counterstrategies in place, here's what it looks like:

- You spend a lot of time feeling frustrated, resentful, and with dwindling hope that you'll ever be able to make peace with food or your body. You wish you had it easier like you think others do, perhaps fantasizing that someone, somewhere gets to lead a life of all the yummiest foods and little physical activity while also enjoying good health and vitality.

- You judge many of your efforts at change as insufficient, thus discouraging yourself from making them. You tend to assume that good nutrition takes more time and energy than you can spare, and that it's too confusing to get right anyway.

- You think backwards about the factors that affect your health and wellbeing the most, feeling attracted to choices that actually put you at medical risk, reduce your quality of life, and guarantee a perpetual sense of unrest. You tend to forget what feeling really good is like, settling more and more for the fleeting enjoyment you get from the very foods that put you in this unfortunate predicament to begin with.

- You keep trying to solve these problems by tackling the most obvious symptom rather than addressing its source. You repeatedly experience negative overall results by doing more of the same even though the same has never worked, long-term. You periodically tire enough of this to give up altogether until the consequences are once again too severe to ignore, then the cycle repeats.

- You feel impatient with how long it takes for change to start feeling more natural and desirable to you. Because it takes longer than you hope, you think more and more that it's not possible at all, giving you yet another reason to quit striving toward a better life.

- You have unrealistic expectations about the ideal body you should be rewarded with if you do the right things, causing you to reject the vastly improved body that you actually do get when you hang in there long enough to achieve it. Though you feel better and enjoy life a great deal more at such times, you overlook those benefits by focusing instead on your disappointment with some aspect of your appearance or the fact that your weight isn't what you'd hoped for. Because you don't appreciate the improved quality of life you have achieved, you don't work to protect it. It slips away again every time.

- You periodically try to spur yourself into healthier behaviors by focusing on goals that you think should motivate you, even though you know they really don't. You criticize yourself for not wanting the "right" goals, rather than figuring out goals that would actually work for you.

- Your network of friends and family includes many people with the same food struggles that you have. When you consider new patterns, it changes the ways that you spend time with those you care about; this can feel uncomfortable and even unsettle some relationships a bit. Due to your own discomfort or pressure from those who don't share your goals, you choose preserving your relationships over improving your health, overlooking ways that you might manage both together.

The demoralizing experience described above is a reasonable description of the lives currently being lived by too many of us. It starts with a distorted sense of what constitutes normal, then continues with a set of perceptions, beliefs, and choices that all lead to feeling hopeless about change.

Life does not have to be this way.

It will be though, if you continue to rely on reflexive beliefs and strategies that don't work for the world in which you live. Most of what you see described above can be improved dramatically by changes that are entirely in your control—and *only* in your control—to make.

The only partial exception is the issue of falling out of step with your friends and family, and even that can be mitigated to some degree by being more proactive with communication and more creative about how you spend time with them.

Distorted beliefs and perceptions can be corrected. Ineffective strategies can be replaced with better ones. This world and this life *can* be successfully navigated. As soon as you start letting go of what's not working anyway, things can get better.

Part Four

Building a Stronger Base for Your Future

Chapter 22
Our Need for Reward: The Key to It All

As discussed in Chapter 19, you are far more likely to maintain personal change for the long term if it is linked to goals that have great emotional importance to you. Most of us will find it challenging to maintain our day-to-day focus on working toward even the most carefully selected goals, however, because we are continually distracted by the emotional brain's insistence on more immediate rewards.

Your emotional brain has the power to turn your life upside down if it feels sufficiently dissatisfied, so it behooves you to keep its needs well met at all times. This will keep it receptive to input from your cortex, a necessary condition of your thriving happily in the modern world.

You need to supply your emotional brain with enough reward to make the present worthwhile, and to do it in a manner that complements your work toward the long-term goals that will create a rewarding future. You need to achieve all of this in ways that minimize negative outcomes, since those detract from total reward value.

Perhaps you can now see why overeating is such a failed strategy for trying to achieve reward for the emotional brain. It produces pleasant sensations that last mere moments, followed shortly after by physical and/or emotional discomfort that lasts for hours, all while setting the stage for potentially dire health consequences to be suffered for years later on. If your aim is to have the most enjoyment in life that you can, overeating is clearly not the way to do it.

Toward a Better Reward System

What your emotional brain seeks—comfort, relief, and reward—is healthy and life-affirming. Every creature with an emotional brain has these needs; they are foundational to life on this planet. You may believe that achieving greater self-control will mean getting better at overcoming or ignoring them, but nothing could be further from the truth. Your long-term success actually depends on meeting them more reliably and effectively than you ever have, and on continuing to do so for life. When you do that, the emotional energy associated with these needs will augment your efforts rather than sabotaging them.

Your emotional brain pulls toward certain choices because those options seem the most rewarding in the moment, and your emotional brain can't see further ahead than that. In order to reward yourself in ways that can compete successfully with the reward you expect to get from eating, you must take into account the innate tendencies of the emotional brain. When using that information as a basis for describing what makes a system of rewards effective, two points stand out.

- The emotional brain must get rewards reliably enough to keep it satisfied in the present. That's what it's going after with a lot of your overeating, so you'll need to fill that vacuum in other ways in order to feel emotionally okay as you practice new eating patterns.

  As personally important as your long-term goals may be, they lack the immediacy to keep your emotional brain consistently motivated. While your cortex knows that great benefits will come from staying the course, your emotional brain just isn't able to wait around that long for a payoff. It needs to be kept taken care of *now*, or at least, very soon.

- Rewards must have sufficient value to *feel* worthwhile. For example, if you are holding a five dollar bill in your hand and I expect you to give it up, I've got to offer you something worth at least as much or you'll have no reason to make the trade. If I offer you a ten dollar bill, that's an obvious trade because you're coming out ahead, but that's not the only trade that will work. If I offer an alternative that's *worth* five dollars to you, you'll be willing to make the trade because you're not losing value in the deal.

This idea of different-but-at-least-equivalent value is a critical concept. Your emotional brain wants a life of sufficient reward and that reward can consist of any combination of things that are worthwhile to you, as long as there's enough total value overall. You might be heavily dependent on food for your reward needs at the moment, but it doesn't have to be that way. Other rewards will do just fine, and having enough of them is the secret to being satisfied with eating differently than you do now.

You have two general types of rewards to consider: external and internal. There are significant differences between them which must be understood if you are to make the best use of each in the system of personal rewards that you ultimately create.

External Rewards

External rewards[1] are so named because they originate outside of you. We are powerfully motivated toward them because there are some—like food, water, and shelter—that we must have at some bare minimum in order to survive at all. External rewards beyond those required for basic survival increase comfort and enjoyment in life, so we like to have more of them when we can get them.

Familiar external rewards in the modern world include the paycheck workers receive for showing up and doing their jobs adequately, or the special treats and privileges that parents use to reward their children for behaving well. External rewards may also be less tangible, like the praise, affection, or trust of others.

External rewards aren't just about being paid off by others for good behavior, however. Think about how rewarding it feels to come in from the cold, or to fall into a comfy bed at the end of a tiring day. For that matter, consider the simple delight of discovering that a package you've been waiting for has arrived sooner than you expected.

These are all pleasant experiences that exist independently of whether or not you've met anyone's expectations; because they come to you from the outside, they are external rewards.

External rewards are wonderful, but they come with limitations. First and foremost, you must have access to the source of the reward in the first place. You can't get a paycheck if you can't find a job, for example. You can't get the affection or admiration of others if you don't have or make the time to invest in those relationships. Nor can you come in from the cold or fall into a comfy bed if you can't afford a decent place to live.

External rewards, since they come from outside of you, are contingent on your access to someone or something that can provide them. If you lack access, you're out of luck.

Reliability is also an issue with external rewards because they are affected by many variables that are out of your control. For example, you might find a job and perform it perfectly, yet still get no paycheck this month if your employer happens to run into serious financial problems. You might do your best to gain someone's trust, only to discover that they are incapable of giving it. Or you might place your order so that you'll definitely get your package in time, but severe weather conditions could delay your shipment anyway. There are countless reasons that, despite making all the right moves, your anticipated reward won't always come.

Food is an external reward, of course. One that—in the developed world—is now highly accessible and reliable, available to most of us far in excess of what we need for survival. The fact that we love food would make it a great reward except that when we eat much more of it than we really need, we subtract from its total reward value by incurring unpleasant physical and emotional costs.

Maximizing our reward from food means having enough of it to meet our physical needs and to have an enjoyable experience, but not so much that bad things—feeling out of control, getting uncomfortably full, adding to health risks—might start to happen. This is all that moderation really means. Eat as much as you can so long as you create only desirable results when you do; stop before you cross the line of "too much" and start giving back some of the reward by bringing on unwanted results.

Eating in this manner guarantees the most possible enjoyment from what we *eat*, but is likely to leave the emotional brain feeling shortchanged if we don't maintain our customary *total* level of reward in some additional ways. If the emotional brain is to accept eating differently for a lifetime, it's going to need some other worthwhile rewards to take the place of all that extra food.

Though it isn't the most effective approach, most people attempt to fill the gap with other external rewards like new clothing or special nights out, especially when certain milestones in weight loss have been achieved. Many, struggling as they are with the diet-induced deprivation of the emotional brain, reward themselves for weight loss with *trigger food*—"I've lost 25 pounds, so I'm going to celebrate with my favorite ice cream!" This, by the way, is one sure sign of an emotional brain that has been neglected and is staging for a full takeover at some point, using the milestone celebration as a warmup.

People engaged in weight-loss projects tend to be very dependent on several less tangible kinds of external rewards as well, most famous among these being the measurement of their weight. Seeing the number on the scale go down is tremendously rewarding and invigorating. It has helped many people to power through significant amounts of weight loss, but there are three drawbacks to reliance on this as a primary reward.

First, there's the reliability problem. Most clients I've worked with have, at one time or another, come into my office and said something like, "I had a *great* week. I ate really well and didn't miss a day of exercise. I felt wonderful and was really proud of myself. Then I got on the scale and it hadn't changed, and I wondered why I'm doing all of this if I'm not getting any results."

Your weight, due to the vagaries of physiology, won't always respond to your efforts in the way that you expect. Many people, upon encountering this particular disappointment, experience at least momentary thoughts of just giving up; a significant number of them actually follow through. It's hazardous to use readings on the scale as a reward if being disappointed by what you see can plunge you headlong into a bout of self-destructive behavior.

Another drawback of using weigh-ins as your primary reward is that most people begin defining "results" exclusively in terms of weight change. Note that in the example above, having a great week and feeling wonderful—experiences anyone in their right mind would always desire—apparently do not count as results worth keeping. The scale is not working well for you if you become so fixated on its readings that you're willing to devalue meaningful and enjoyable benefits just because they're not accompanied by the number that you wanted.

The third drawback to reliance on the scale for reward is that even if all goes exactly as you hope and plan, the numbers will only go down until you reach your goal weight. Then what? Will you get the same thrill out of seeing the same, healthy number day after day that you used to get from watching the number regularly going down? Falling numbers may provide the reward to help you get down to where you want to be, at least temporarily, but what's going to provide the reward that keeps you there once you've arrived?

Another less tangible external reward that boosts many people through some period of greater self-control with food is the acclaim they get from others as they start to look healthier and more fit, i.e., "Wow, you're looking great! What you're doing is incredible!"

While some people feel resentful about this—*Why didn't you think I was important before I lost weight?*—many enjoy it and ride the wave of enthusiasm with continued focus and success. As with the scale though, that which powers you through weight loss may not come through for you in sustaining it long-term.

People notice weight loss because it's novel; you're different and you're continuing to change. If you are fortunate enough to eventually stabilize at a lower, healthier weight, that means you'll stop changing and the state of your health and appearance will gradually become less interesting to others.

The regular chorus of, "Wow, you're looking great," will become a far less regular and smaller chorus of, "Wow, you're *still* looking great," over time as people get used to it and focus their attention elsewhere. If you've been heavily reliant on the acclaim of others as a reward for your efforts, this could be a problem when it comes to maintaining at a steady state going forward.

External rewards are an essential part of our lives. We need some of them to survive and beyond the level of basic necessity, having more of them makes life a lot nicer. They certainly have their place in the grand scheme of things.

When it comes to keeping your emotional brain happy while you're changing your relationship with food, however, you're best advised to use external rewards in conjunction with something more accessible, reliable, powerful, and lasting.

Internal Rewards

Internal rewards[2] are enjoyable emotions which are generated inside of you, and you've probably experienced many of them without really thinking of them as such. It has happened each time you've felt amused, relaxed, pleasantly surprised, deeply moved, peaceful, delighted, content, grateful, hopeful, confident, appreciated, loved, excited, or intrigued.

It has happened when you've felt important to others, or even when you've simply felt appreciated. It has happened when you've felt good about seeing someone you care about experience a personal success or sidestep a potential health threat.

It is an internal reward to be faced with a challenge that is invigorating, inspiring, or fascinating. It's an additional reward when you discover that a challenge has brought out more from you than you knew you had. If all goes well, this can lead to the reward of feeling satisfied by a job well done, or at least with having made an admirable effort.

It is rewarding to have a sense of meaning, a sense of purpose, to feel that your time has been well spent, or that your efforts have amounted to something worthwhile. It can even be an internal reward to get some unwanted task over with so that it is now behind you, rather than in front of you.

Internal rewards feel so good that you may find it somewhat rewarding simply to read the examples above and briefly recall times when you've had feelings like those described.

When you want to do something for its own sake without need of external rewards, you are doing it for the internal rewards. When someone says, "If they weren't paying me to do this, I'd do it for free," that person is describing work that provides internal rewards that exceed the value of the paycheck that comes with it.

Some external rewards make life possible, while others make it enjoyable. It is the internal rewards, however, that make life fulfilling. When it comes to true depth of personal satisfaction, internal rewards are the key.

Eating is highly enjoyable, but it is primarily about external rewards. You might disbelieve this at first because you probably have many treasured memories of wonderful meals shared with others, for example, which may cause you to think of eating as more emotionally valuable than it actually is. The reality is that these memories are treasured not because of how good the food was or even how much fun it was to eat it, but because of whom you were with at the time.

It's the internal reward of bonding with loved ones—not the external reward of the food itself—that gives such memories their well-earned emotional charge. If you have any doubt about this, try replaying one of those memories in your mind right now with one important change: the people are gone, and it's just you and the food. Even if the food is great and you'd still enjoy eating it alone, chances are *that* memory would never rise to any real importance in the bigger story of your life.

By all means, keep your warm memories close to your heart, but be clear about where the significance really lies so that you don't credit eating with more emotional power than it could possibly have. This more objective perspective will help you to feel better about considering some changes in how you eat, and to discover for yourself that such changes don't cause anything of real emotional importance to be lost.

With the superior emotional value of internal rewards now clearly in mind, you may begin to appreciate how powerful a role they can play in your personal reward system. Internal rewards consist of good feelings, and good feelings are what your emotional brain craves the most, despite how easily it can get distracted by the cheap, external fix of food.

Turning to food for emotional reasons—whether to get good feelings or to alleviate bad ones—often results in eating too much. This happens in part simply because the emotional reward available from food is so superficial that we try to compensate by eating a lot more of it. Unfortunately, a bunch of cheap fixes don't add up to one good one.

Given that overeating adds to problems rather than alleviating them, using food for emotional reasons also means that you'll often end up in greater need of emotional relief than when you started. Until you understand this cycle, you are destined to keep returning to food for something it can't give you. It would be great for all of us if food *could* create real, lasting emotional serenity, but it can't. It's just food.

Internal rewards, on the other hand, are quite effective in this regard and also have some very desirable qualities. They are constantly available because the capacity for them is within you at all times, and they create no unwanted consequences. You don't need to have enough money to afford them or extra time to carry them out, and you're not dependent on anyone or anything outside of yourself to make them possible.

Internal rewards are the key to keeping your emotional brain content so that your cortex can carry on with creating the best life possible from what's available to you. If you remember nothing else about internal rewards, remember this: they feel good.

You'll be hard-pressed to identify many food experiences that provide anything near the satisfaction you can get from even the simplest of internal rewards. Using them more intentionally may not come naturally at first, but it is a skill that can be cultivated over time. The better you get at it, the happier you'll be.

Make Each Day Worthwhile

You can only reach and maintain your goals if the whole process feels worthwhile as you do it, so the point of an effective reward system is to keep your emotional brain safely and reliably satisfied, day after day. This creates desirable life experiences in the present while paving the way toward a healthy and enjoyable future. The best reward system will use a combination of internal and external rewards that are dependable, realistic, and worthwhile, fueling motivation that lasts for a lifetime.

Chapter 23
Using Rewards to Drive Results

The key to creating a self-sustaining system of ongoing reward is to set up daily goals that are completely doable. Each time one of these goals is completed, it provides two internal rewards: an immediate sense of accomplishment, plus the feeling of real progress toward any longer-term goals you have.

This means that you get to enjoy rewarding feelings every day rather than waiting for a single, big payoff at the end. This is especially important for goals that will take months or years to realize, because time frames of that magnitude can feel so discouraging that you might sometimes be tempted to give up.

The Power of Breaking It Down
Once you've identified a long-term goal to which you aspire, the next thing you'll need to do is break it down into its component parts. These, in turn, will help you identify the day-to-day actions that will eventually make it real.

While the goal itself may feel grand, distant, and hard to imagine, the individual steps required to achieve it are simple and clearly defined. This is important because your project has to feel both real and possible to you if you are to sustain your efforts over time.

Take the example of earning a high school diploma. This typically takes *12 years*—an astoundingly long project time by anyone's definition—but few of us look at it as a whole. Instead, we tend to look at it one year at a time. Within each individual year, we concentrate on doing well in each grading period, one at a time. Within each grading period, we concentrate on completing each of the required assignments and tests, one at a time. To succeed on each assignment and test, we concentrate on the daily work of going to class and studying. If you take the overall goal and break it all the way down, you get a pyramid structure that looks as follows:

High School Diploma

12 years of education

Dozens of grading periods

Hundreds of assignments and tests

Daily tasks: attend class, study, do homework

Getting a high school education is a huge, vague, intimidating concept involving a span of time no one can really grasp; it's an amazing accomplishment, especially when you consider that it is routinely accomplished by *children*. The reason so many perfectly ordinary individuals manage to do it is that they keep their focus on the manageable requirements of a single day—they just do it many, many times. Few people could bear the prospect of going to school for 12 years, but most can handle the prospect of going to school *today*.

That's the power of breaking big goals down into smaller segments. It keeps you focused on simple, specific actions that are within your control and abilities, and it keeps you focused on the present, the only moment in which it is ever possible to act. It also provides the reassurance that if you have an off day, your next opportunity for success is right around the corner.

Personal effectiveness is always about keeping your focus on what you can do in this moment that will contribute the most to the outcome you seek. This is convenient, given that this moment also happens to be all your emotional brain can focus on anyway. It's no coincidence that "one day at a time" is a core concept for anyone in recovery from an addiction. One day at a time is all any of us can ever do, whether we realize it or not. When we keep our attention on the best action we can take in any given moment, we can accomplish amazing things.

Before you start breaking your longer-term personal goal down into the daily actions that will make it a reality, it is important to realize the true nature of any goal that pertains to your ongoing wellbeing: it is, by definition, *ongoing*. Many goals in life are of the once-and-done variety, like paying off a car loan, painting a room, or planning your next vacation. These are the kinds of goals that, once reached, require no further effort or attention because there is nothing more to do.

When it comes to goals that involve changing your health, your abilities, or your personal practices, however, you must realize that these are not projects with finish lines. Your freshly painted room won't unpaint itself just because you stop thinking about it once you've gotten it done, but your improved quality of life will definitely begin to unravel if you don't keep doing the things that made it possible in the first place. One day at a time is the way you create change, and also the way you *keep* it—just one day, involving simple choices that you are completely equipped to make. That's all you ever have to do.

Breaking Down Health-Related Goals
The pyramid structure that supports any health-related goal consists of these layers:

GOAL

The transformation
that makes the goal
possible

The new patterns that create the
necessary transformation

The daily practices that build the new patterns
and then keep them in place

If your goal was attainable today, you'd already have reached it. Anything you define as a goal, then, is something that is not possible for you yet, but which you hope to have in the future. If you want something that is not possible yet, that means you will have to become different in some meaningful way—you will need to transform—so that the goal can become a reality. Transformations do not occur as a result of wishful thinking (unfortunately), so you will need to change some fundamental aspects of how you live—create some new patterns—in order for the necessary transformation to occur. That brings us to the foundation layer of the structure, the things you do on a daily basis that drive the construction of the rest of the pyramid. Your foundation layer will be customized according to your own needs, but if your goal involves any aspect of your health or physical capability, it will always include some focus on nutrition and body conditioning. Here's one example, previously mentioned in Chapter 19:

Ability to play on the floor with kids

Become stronger, more flexible, and able to rise unassisted from the flloor.

Exercise and stretch more; eat to increase energy and reduce inflammation.

Daily: 20-minute walk or 10-minute strength workout (alternate each day); stretch for five minutes; eat mostly whole food in healthy portions.

Disclaimer: The figure above is an example, <u>not a recommendation</u>. Always consult your doctor for a plan that is appropriate to both your goal and your personal medical status.

Using the example above, if you can't play on the floor with kids today but wish to become someone who can, you need to transform. You'll need to become stronger, more flexible, and more able to rise independently than the person you are today. In order to become and remain that more able person, you'll need to do some things differently, involving new patterns in how you approach physical activity and food.

Though any health-related goal will involve basic, effective self-care, the daily tasks will vary depending on the nature of the goal. Here's how the pyramid might look if your goal is to get fit enough to be able to have fun on an adventure vacation:

**Increase fitness
for an adventure
vacation**

Have more strength
and stamina; be able
to walk/stand for
several hours daily.

More walking and other exercise;
eat to increase energy and reduce
inflammation.

Daily: 30-40 minutes of exercise targeted to
increase muscle strength, aerobic capacity, or
walking range (different focus each day); eat
mostly whole foods in healthy portions.

Disclaimer: The figure above is an example, not a recommendation. Always consult your doctor for a plan that is appropriate to both your goal and your personal medical status.

Each of the goals detailed above involves improving fitness, self-care, and dietary quality, but the second goal requires significantly greater physical ability. As a result, the daily practices for the second goal are more challenging, requiring more time and effort. If you want to be able to participate in an active vacation but you do only the daily practices associated with being able to play on the floor with kids, you will not meet your goal.

The beauty of creating a pyramid specific to your personal goal is that it shows you exactly what you need to do in order to get what you want, and why. This is how to get your emotional brain on board so that its power fuels your efforts instead of undermining them.

You may note that the foundation of pyramids like these, where the tasks are simple and clearly defined, is the only level where you ever have any work to do. Do what's necessary there and the remaining layers will build themselves.

This process works for any long-term goal, but is still useful even if you haven't been able to identify one yet. Just set your sights on a simple benefit or improvement that you know you'd enjoy, and which you know you could achieve if you worked toward it consistently for a month or two. Perhaps it's getting back into an uncomfortably snug piece of clothing that you miss. It could be a simple physical ability that is *just* out of your reach at the moment, but which you could recover fairly quickly if you focused on getting it back. Or maybe you'd just like to be able to get up a flight of stairs without feeling terrible by the time you get to the top.

Whatever it is, the small daily tasks that will bring it to you will involve some measure of improving your nutrition and working your body more purposefully. It's a lot easier to value those efforts when you can see a near-future payoff that will result in some obvious improvement to your life experience.

Once you get that first payoff, you're likely to notice that something else you'd like has now moved a bit closer—not quite in reach, but close enough to look doable with an additional month or two of focus. You may find that you can just pull yourself along, one minor improvement at a time, always focusing on whatever else you'd like next that would make your life a bit more enjoyable.

If you do have a longer-term goal, constructing a pyramid like those above will show you exactly how your daily practices relate to the goal you care about. You'll also be able to see very clearly that your goal can't possibly happen with*out* those practices. Simple actions like taking a walk or eating a good breakfast—done one day at a time—have the power to change your life.

Once you've determined some useful daily actions that will move you toward your goal, it's easy to monitor your progress in terms of a simple, daily to-do list. If you've created an effective list for the day, the items on it will be clearly defined; they will be easy to do and it will be obvious to you whether or not you're doing what is necessary to achieve what you want.

Each time you complete an item on your list, you get the internal rewards of achievement for the day, progress for the future, and an increasing sense that you are able to create good results. An example of one day's objectives might look like this:

- ✓ Have a quick bowl of whole-grain cereal for breakfast.
- ✓ Take an enjoyable, nutritious snack to have at work; avoid snack machines.
- ✓ Walk for 20 minutes.
- ✓ Stand up most of the time during phone calls.
- ✓ Drink more water and less diet soda.

A list like this helps you to stay focused on the one thing you can control—the choices you make today—while reminding you that the requirements for success are quite manageable. There will seldom be a reason to miss your objectives for the day as long as you've set them up in a way that is acceptable to your emotional brain.

This is where customization of the foundation layer of the pyramid comes into play. We all have to support the same key elements of self-care, but we can each do it in ways that fit the best with our personal goals, individual circumstances, and emotional needs. One size does not fit all. Another to-do list, completely different from the one above, yet equally useful:

- ✓ Have a salad as part of at least one meal.
- ✓ Take a few minutes to set up easy, nutritious food options for tomorrow.
- ✓ Do stretches and light exercises while watching TV.
- ✓ Sit for no more than 20 minutes at a time all day.
- ✓ Substitute air-popped popcorn for manufactured snacks.

Or this:

- ✓ Limit evening screen time to a maximum of two hours.
- ✓ Chop salad veggies for the week or prep ingredients for tomorrow's dinner.
- ✓ Eat treat foods only if doing nothing else at the same time.
- ✓ Use small dishes and bowls to limit portion size naturally.
- ✓ Take stairs rather than elevators, and walk the longer way around when possible.

Lists like these—which will probably have some core items that repeat each day, along with a few that vary from day to day depending on your schedule and circumstances—help you to create better outcomes more reliably and to stay mentally focused on your mission even as other distractions arise. Having such a list, even if it's only in your head, gives you an easy way to monitor how you're doing at getting to all of the items before the end of each day. Having the list in print is a real boost for those who get a little shot of internal satisfaction from checking off things as they go.

You will increase your internal rewards significantly by simply pausing to notice your achievements as they occur: *I nailed the list today and it wasn't even that hard. I can do this.* A feeling of accomplishment is one of the most potent internal rewards there is, so you'll want to assure that you take advantage of every opportunity to enjoy it!

Meaningful change is achieved one small act at a time and each one you complete is the opportunity for a nice set of immediate internal rewards, but there's something simple you can do to amplify your rewards even more.

Research shows that those who make a point of focusing on the small wins along the way experience 22% higher life satisfaction than those who focus only on the big prize at the end.[1] Doable daily goals give you a reliable source of those small wins. They also help you to build habits that make you stronger and more effective as you move steadily closer to your long-term goals.

Persistence is the key to most accomplishments, but we can only muster it if we are working toward something that we want and which we believe to be possible. Therefore, the practices you choose must have obvious relevance to a goal you care about, and you must believe that you are capable of them—these are the keys to maintaining motivation and hope.

Persistence means that you just keep showing up and stubbornly doing what you can, refusing to quit. You might be interested to know that persistent people tend to practice certain mental strategies that are available to all of us. They spend a lot of time thinking about what they have managed to achieve so far, using their success-to-date to propel them forward into each new step. They frequently remind themselves that what they seek to do *can* be done, and that they are capable of doing it.[2] These are empowering, self-motivating habits of thought that anyone can practice.

Chances are you've already experienced some occasion in life in which you just wouldn't give up, no matter what. It might have involved something you are passionate about or someone who is very important to you. Maybe something just got you feeling really stubborn. Whatever it was, you knew you wouldn't take no for an answer and you doggedly stayed the course until you achieved your objective. You probably felt strong and effective when you did this, because persistence can be quite satisfying that way. The key to unleashing it within yourself is to assure that you have emotional brain buy-in every step of the way.

You are capable of the base-of-the-pyramid actions that make amazing things possible. You are. As long as you remember that and keep appreciating the value of each small step you take, you can enjoy a steady stream of internal rewards while making your life a little better every single day. You may sometimes find your efforts tiring, but with your emotional brain agreeably on board, you'll never find them burdensome.

More Rewards—Focusing on Progress

Focusing on the small wins of each day generates a lot of internal reward, but you can build upon that even further by occasionally stepping back to appreciate the change that is gradually occurring in your life as a result of your efforts:

- Look at how your practices of today compare to those of a month ago, three months ago, or even all the way back to when you first started experimenting with change.

- Notice how you're gradually feeling more in control with food, more of the time. Remember how often you used to overeat to the point of shame, regret, and physical discomfort; notice how much more you enjoy yourself now.

- Notice how you're planning ahead more now for your eating, and how this creates experiences that you later look back on with gratitude rather than regret.

- Notice how your body is getting stronger, more comfortable, and more reliable for you.

- Notice how you can move with greater ease and confidence.

- Notice how you hurt less than you used to (both physically and emotionally).

- Notice how you are beginning to fit a little better into the various physical spaces of your life.

- Notice the options that are beginning to open up to you as your health, strength, and focus improve. Think about how much more enjoyable your life will become as new options continue to become available to you.

- Notice that you're learning how to use nutritious food to create meals that are enjoyable to anticipate, see, smell, and eat—one savory, fully noticed bite at a time—yet which don't trigger you into losing control.

- Notice how relaxing it is to eat with content control. Notice how this compares to the intense internal struggles you used to have so much more of the time.

- Notice the hope and personal effectiveness you feel now compared to how you felt at first.

- Look at the progress you've made toward your goal compared to when you began.

When you do these periodic reviews, <u>always</u> beware the natural tendency to fall back into all-or-nothing thinking (Chapter 13). You'll notice it in thoughts like these:

Yeah, but that's not enough.

It's taking too long.

That's nice, but it's a drop in the bucket. This will take forever, if I even get there at all.

I should be seeing more results than this.

I've lost weight way faster than this before. Maybe I should go back on a diet.

I've got a big problem, and big problems require big solutions. These little daily things I'm doing couldn't possibly be enough to make a dent in this.

Every important accomplishment in life consists of many small, interim steps. Don't let all-or-nothing thinking fool you into believing they are unimportant when, in fact, they are the *only* path to long-term success.

If you focus consistently on your new daily practices for a month and *don't* notice any progress of the types described above, it means one (or both) of two things.

First, you might be so unaccustomed to this kind of personal evaluation that you have trouble doing it enough to notice the changes you are, in fact, creating. If that's the case, it can help to compare notes with a trusted friend (who exhibits no tendencies toward sabotage) to get some objective outside feedback.

If someone knows you well and cares about you, they're likely to notice as you become calmer, happier, more focused, and more effective, even if they can't quite say why. If they tell you that you just seem better in some hard-to-describe way, that's enough confirmation for you to know your actions are having an effect. Your challenge then will be to get better at noticing your results yourself so that you can enjoy them more fully.

Journaling can be a good way to help with this. If you take notes of your experience along the way, you'll eventually find yourself reading old notes that describe things you'd completely forgotten about, but which now give you much better perspective on today. The more you practice this, the better you'll get at being able to do it purely in thought if you prefer. Frankly, though, seeing your progress in a journal is another potent reward. There's nothing quite like seeing a visible record of how far you've come to help you appreciate the reality of it.

The second reason you may not notice any progress is that you might not actually be making any. If that's the case, it shows that you've either been a lot less consistent than you thought, or that you've whittled your daily objectives down to the point where they are too small to create meaningful change.

It's been my experience that most people know whether or not they're making an honest effort. If you're finding it hard to get motivated, you have fallen into the old trap of trying to move forward without making the process worthwhile for your emotional brain. In that case, you'll need to dig back in and look some more for what will work to fuel your efforts for change. If you can't manage this on your own or with friends, then it might help to consult with a counselor who can help you sort it out.

On the other hand, if you *are* putting your heart into it and are failing to get the kinds of results you see described above, it might be a good idea to schedule a checkup with your doctor. There could be some underlying medical issue that is getting in your way, which will keep you stuck until it is identified and addressed. What could be more demoralizing than doing all the right things for the right reasons, yet having little come of it? That shouldn't happen, so if it is happening to you, it means something is wrong. Get whatever help you need so that you can get on with moving forward.

Yet *More* Rewards—The Power of Gratitude

The emotional brain needs reward—a lot of it, and frequently—in order to feel okay. Many of us have distilled our life experience down to trying to meet our reward quota almost entirely with food. This chapter so far has been about how you can trade some external food rewards for more powerful internal rewards as you take control of yourself and your life, but even that still frames the concept of reward in overly narrow terms. There is so much more.

Imagine living a life of poverty. Now imagine that you actually have a million dollars available to you (perhaps a wealthy relative left you an inheritance) but you don't know it (nobody from that wing of the family knows you, so they can't find you).

You are technically a millionaire, but in reality, you are quite poor. As long as you remain unaware of your windfall, it's the same as not having it at all. Imagine the stress of living day to day, not knowing if you'll ever be able to relax and feel okay. Imagine how desperately your emotional brain would crave relief—any relief—to escape the burden of always struggling to meet your most basic needs.

Now imagine how your feelings would change if only you knew about the money ...

Many of us live in a manner that is surprisingly similar, though the contrast is less extreme. Whatever the challenges of our life situations, we are all constantly surrounded by reasons to be grateful, but many of us fail to notice it for days, weeks, even years at a time. Some of us never notice it at all. A pitifully small sampling:

- Do you have somewhere comfortable, dry, and safe to sleep at night?

- Do you have easy access to water that is safe to drink?

- Do you get to take warm baths or showers whenever you want to?

- Can you get enough food to prevent you from ever feeling painfully, frighteningly hungry?

- Do you have transportation that allows you to operate in a world larger than the distance you can walk from your home?

- Do you have clothing and footwear that allow you to stay protected and reasonably comfortable in a variety of weather conditions?

If you are fortunate enough to be able to answer *yes* to any of the items on this list, it's probably been some time since you've stopped to marvel at how lucky you are to have them. Imagine how different your life would be without any one of them. Imagine how much better you would feel if you remained more consciously aware of what you have going for you.

Instead, most of us spend a lot of our time frustrated, concerned, and irritated over *so* many things—most of them quite fleeting—while remaining essentially blind to the many advantages of our lives. Think about the toll this takes on the emotional brain—this insistent sense of, *I'm not okay. In fact, I'm not okay in a dozen different ways every day. I'm not sure I'll ever be okay.*

A distressed emotional brain will become increasingly desperate and undiscriminating in its attempts to get relief. The more stressful you find your life to be, the more likely you are to make short-sighted choices as you try to help yourself feel better. If you focus a lot on the disappointments and problems in your life—complaining rather than taking constructive action—you will maximize the distress you feel, thus also maximizing your need for cheap, easy relief.

The solution to this self-defeating cycle is to look at your life situation with fresh eyes, focusing more on the many reasons you have to be grateful; the list above is a simple start. Seriously, if you have advantages like adequate clothing, a place to live, safe water, enough food, and reliable transportation, that is cause for deep, enthusiastic gratitude. Just ask anyone who *doesn't* have those things.

If you never take a moment to ponder your amazing good fortune, you are little different than the clueless millionaire. If you do take a moment, and do so regularly, you'll be able to tap into a vast supply of both internal and external rewards for your emotional brain that have been hiding in plain sight all along—they're already *right there.* You don't have to do anything to reap these rewards other than to *notice* them. You can't find an easier source of reward than that.

Periodic reminders of how much you have to be grateful for are very comforting to the emotional brain: *I'm okay, and lots of things are in place to help me stay that way.* While this alone is unlikely to make your food urges vanish, it can certainly quiet them down a bit. It is no coincidence that cultivating an "attitude of gratitude" figures prominently in so many recovery programs. Gratitude helps you to feel better, keep a more balanced perspective, and manage your life more effectively. It reduces the distress that might tilt your emotional brain into self-destructive strategies for seeking relief, and acts as a multiplier for every reward available to you.

The Day-to-Day Purpose of Your Long-Term Goal

The first thing a long-term goal will do for you is help to get the ball rolling. Since a goal is something you want but don't yet have, and which you won't get unless you start doing something different, establishing one helps you to feel more open to the possibility of change.

Your long-term goal will next help you—when you detail its pyramid—to break down what you want into increasingly simpler units of action that occur within the space of each day. Because you see there are actions that you can take within a timeframe you can manage, a goal sets the stage for many interim rewards in addition to inspiring optimism and hope.

From that point forward, your goal becomes a clear litmus test that you can apply to each of your daily choices: *Does this get me closer to my goal, move me further away from it, or keep me in the same place?* Ideally, most of your choices will be small steps in the direction you've chosen. Some will result in holding steady where you are, because that's the flow of life—sometimes you move forward and sometimes you rest. As long as you're not resting so much that you can't get anywhere, it's all part of the process.

While some amount of rest is necessary and healthy, some amount of moving in the wrong direction—despite having no upside—is simply to be expected. The important thing is to avoid it as much as possible, contain it quickly when it happens, and focus on discovering whatever lesson has been revealed in the process. Every step in the wrong direction means that you're getting further from your goal rather than closer, and that means you'll have to make up the lost ground before you can get back to making actual progress.

Detours of this type on the way toward your personal goal are not the end of the world when they happen, but it's much, much better when they don't. Just focus on minimizing the damage as quickly as possible when necessary, the sooner to get happily back on your way in the direction that you want.

Chapter 24
Dealing with Unwanted Feelings and Bad Days

Most overeaters use food as their primary defense against uncomfortable emotional states.[1] Whether it is sadness, disappointment, depression, anxiety, frustration, self-doubt, anger, fatigue, feeling "off," being overwhelmed, or simple boredom, food is now the go-to solution for most of us when we don't like how we feel.

Food usually provides the instant hit of reward or relief that the emotional brain seeks, but the experience is fleeting. The emotional brain must then keep going after more and more food, trying to string together many brief rewards in order keep unwanted feelings at bay.

Meanwhile, the problem that triggered those feelings either remains unresolved or gets worse from neglect, even as the eating creates additional problems that will generate *more* unwanted feelings. The vicious downward spiral is that the worse you feel, the more you want to escape through food, but the more you escape through food, the more you maintain or even aggravate the conditions that made you feel bad in the first place.

What to do?

Your Life as a Table
The best defense against bad days and unwanted feelings is to have fewer of them in the first place, and there is no better way to accomplish that than to live a balanced lifestyle.

The easiest way I've found to understand the concept of balanced living is to think of a table as a metaphor for your life. The structure is supported by the legs beneath which—in the case of your life—can vary greatly in number and type. Common examples of such legs are shown in the list that follows.

Factors that Affect Life Balance and Stability

- Each *very* close loved one
- Parenting
- Intimate partnership
- Extended family
- Pets
- Each important life goal
- Any personal passion
- Community involvement
- Social groups
- Employment
- School
- Spiritual practices
- Health
- Volunteering
- Hobbies

Together, legs like these keep your life stable and strong. A table supported by three or four legs is far steadier than a table with only one or two, and so it is with your life. People with several good legs to rely on have much greater buffering against the vicissitudes of life than do those with fewer options.

If you are a person whose whole life is your job, for example—a single leg to stand on—you're vulnerable to experiencing an emotional crisis if a serious job-related problem develops. Imagine your emotional position if you get reassigned or demoted, are given an impossible amount of work to complete, or end up assigned to a boss who bullies you.

Where is your sanctuary when your only source of identity and purpose becomes unreliable or unavailable? How do you recharge, reassess, and find a way to feel okay when there is no other emotional place for you to go? Lacking better options, you are likely to seek relief in short-sighted, desperate ways that make your situation worse instead of better.

Or how about if you've devoted your entire life to your family, neglecting your personal needs and development in the process, only to find that you are now estranged from your spouse as your kids are launching into their own independent lives? What's left for you to stand on?

Now imagine either of these worrisome predicaments, but with the difference that you have supportive friends to talk to, a hobby that helps with stress management, or you take good care of yourself so that you feel stronger and can think more clearly when things go wrong. Better yet, imagine the difference if you have two of these things going for you, or even all three. It's a lot easier to manage a crisis in one part of your life if you've got some other parts you can still count on along the way.

The main point, as always, is to set up your life as well as you can so that your emotional brain always has as many reasons as possible to feel okay. Just as a table with only one or two legs is inherently insecure, far too reliant on good luck in order to remain upright, so are you. If you have only a leg or two to stand on, you're always just one bad turn away from your life becoming unmanageably stressful. When that bad turn comes, your vulnerability will set the stage for regrettable episodes with food.

If you're starting to realize that your life has been balanced on just a precarious leg or two, rest assured that greater stability is nearer than you think. Having two legs to stand on is considerably better than one, yet still leaves you vulnerable because it's not that hard for two legs (job and one significant relationship, for instance) to be compromised at the same time.

Once you get to three legs, however, your emotional security increases dramatically simply because it's so rare for three legs to all weaken or fail at once. For that reason, I recommend doing what you can to get three legs in place if at all possible; an additional one or two never hurts.

This makes for a life that benefits your emotional brain in two important ways. It's a more diversified and interesting life, which is desirable in any event, and having a few strong legs in place gives you more of a safety margin in the event of a setback. Your emotional brain is both happier and safer, and is therefore less inclined to lunge after food for comfort or relief.

It's theoretically possible to gain control with food if you have only one or two well-developed areas of your life, but it's a *lot* easier if you have more. If you—like many people—only have one or two, chances are that health is not one of them. In that case, there are compelling reasons to make health something that you always nurture and prioritize.

First, it's always available to you as an option; regardless of your circumstances, you always have the ability to choose in ways that bolster and protect whatever health you have.

That leads to the second great thing about choosing health, which is that even when the rest of your life is crumbling (we all go through those times), focusing on health gives you a way to keep generating successes and maintain some sense of control, all while positioning yourself to get the rest of your life back in order as soon as possible.

Many people abandon their health when the chips are down. They believe that they lack the time or energy for it in the midst of a crisis, when the reality is that hanging onto your health could be what gets you *through* the crisis. As someone who has relied upon this strategy a number of times myself, I can assure you that it works. I've never seen it fail anyone.

If you add the health leg to your structure and find that you still need another leg or two, I strongly recommend that you try a new hobby or revive an old one. Few of my incoming clients seem to have hobbies, often because they feel too busy and spread too thin to have the time.

This presumes that hobbies are frivolous pursuits meant only for those with time on their hands, which misses an important point. Hobbies, by definition, are something we do *for pleasure*, which is what the emotional brain seeks. If you don't make time for sources of pleasure that enrich your life in the ways that hobbies do, you're more likely to seek cheap pleasure on the run as we do with food.

So by all means, get a hobby, even if it's only for a few minutes here and there; it will bring positive energy to your life while adding considerably to the stability of your life structure.

A balanced lifestyle will keep your emotional brain calm and content more of the time as a matter of course, which will reduce the frequency and intensity of your urges to overeat. This is important since toning the urges down even a little bit will make them more manageable.

It will pay off even more, however, when you are going through difficult times. When emotional unrest occurs in a life of general balance and stability, you have a wide variety of built-in, effective options available for helping yourself when necessary.

When that unrest occurs in a life of precarious balance and disorganization, on the other hand, you have little recourse. The chaos of your life means that you have few helpful options readily available, and also that nothing you do will help for very long in any event; food naturally starts to seem like the only salvation.

Increasing lifestyle balance—if you don't already have it—is an essential part of setting yourself up to have greater control and peace with food.

Non-Food Strategies for Soothing Your Emotional Brain

If food has been your main emotional-management tool for a long time, it may be hard to remember that anything else is possible, but this is actually very easy to challenge. Imagine for a moment that you are experiencing one of those feelings that typically drives you toward food. This time, however, food is simply unavailable—you don't have any, and you can't get any. Nor, for the sake of argument, do you have access to alcohol, drugs, gambling, or any other potentially harmful ways to distract yourself.

So, here you are with the same old crummy feelings you've always tried to escape, but none of the obvious escapes is available. If you are determined to try to find some way to help yourself feel better anyway—coping instead of escaping—what might you do?

When I ask this question of clients, it usually doesn't take them long to start generating ideas—*good* ideas that would not occur to them if the cheap fix of food was readily at hand. It seems that the mere availability of food often stunts our ability to think creatively when it comes to easing emotional unrest. You may well find that this is the case for you.

There are actually many ways to address emotional needs that yield far greater comfort and peace than anything you can get from food. The advantages of healthy, non-food strategies are considerable:

- They help you to feel better and more in control, while food is more likely to make you feel numb and out of control.

- They increase your mental clarity and sense of purpose, whereas food keeps you feeling fogged and lacking direction.

- They create benefits that you can enjoy both in the moment and often for an extended period of time afterwards, while any relief you get from eating is over as soon as you stop.

- They solve problems rather than creating more of them; they make your life better rather than worse.

- Because they effectively calm the emotional brain, they strengthen the cortex. A strongly engaged cortex means you'll live with greater effectiveness and satisfaction in general, as well as being a better problem solver when the need arises.

If you need help getting started, here are some tried-and-true ideas to consider. Each has the potential to be helpful for a variety of challenges, and you'll learn through experimentation which ones tend to help you the most. Some of these suggestions even have the potential to become strong legs in that balanced lifestyle we were just talking about, so it's good to watch for those along the way.

Spend Some Time with People Who Care About You

If you're having an off day or a rough time, it usually helps to reach out to others whom you trust and enjoy—in person, if possible. You'll find the companionship uplifting whether or not you talk about what's bothering you and it's likely to be a far better way to spend the time than just holing up alone with your bad feelings. It can be a reassuring reminder of valued relationships that remain strong as you deal with some other part of your life that may be in need of repair or improvement.

Connecting with those who care about you offers the reassurance that while you may doubt your own value sometimes, they don't. They can continue to see and appreciate the best parts of you even when you can't, and that can help you to remember that those parts exist. That can help.

If you choose to discuss your concerns with them, you may find that others can offer a more objective perspective. This can help you to reconsider your own point of view, which in turn may result in you adopting a more strategic approach toward whatever it is that's troubling you.

Since getting together for meals may be part of your food problem in the first place, it's a good idea to purposely spend time with others in some alternate ways. It may help to try a slightly different version of the question posed earlier: *If we wanted to spend time together and sharing food was not an option, what else could we do?*

Never underestimate the power of something as simple as sharing a walk with a friend on a nice day, for example. You could work together on some home project that one of you needs to finish, or go to an attraction or event that you're both likely to enjoy. Maybe you could try something new together that neither of you has ever done before; that one's a win no matter what, because you'll either find a promising new activity to share in the future or come away with funny stories to tell about why you didn't like it. There are many non-food ways to spend time together that we've forgotten about; you might find it quite energizing for both yourself and your relationships to rediscover them.

When you turn your attention away from your bad feelings and toward a valued relationship, you may find that the simple break from your own solitary, problem-centered thinking is enough to give you a new and more helpful perspective. The fact is that some unwanted feelings have a limited lifespan—they will simply pass without effort on your part if you just occupy yourself in positive ways for long enough. Time spent with a good companion helps that time to pass more quickly, and in a way that brings quality to your life rather than detracting from it.

Do Something Physical

Physical activity is great for reducing stress and clearing the mind, but many of us have lost track of that bit of wisdom in recent decades. If you're in a bad mood of some kind, getting active provides an immediate, concrete alternative for your attention; you focus away from what is bothering you on the inside, and toward something you can do on the outside.

When you do this, you go from spinning in pointless emotional circles to producing some tangible result, whether that is to walk a mile, clean a closet, work out, mow your lawn, or wash your car. At the very least, you've converted your energy into activity that reduces your stress instead of adding to it, which is a big improvement. Becoming productive in the process is a bonus, because feeling productive is internally rewarding in addition to creating results that improve your life situation.

If you pursue your chosen activity with enough attention, you'll give your mind a break that will allow it to reset a bit. You'll be focusing on different thoughts and different actions, possibly in a different setting, all of which will allow you to return to your concern with a fresher and more effective perspective when you're ready.

When you redirect yourself into physical activity for the purpose of managing unwanted feelings, you may or may not feel rewarded by what you're doing once you start. The likelihood is that you'll eventually be glad for having done it, but even if it doesn't work out that way (some moods are pretty tough to break), you'll still be better off for at least making a positive attempt. That in itself has value, because it means you're not quitting. You may not be thriving at the moment, but you're also not giving up. That is a powerful and important message to yourself—one that is always well worth sending

Emotions come in a variety of energy levels. When you're using physical activity as a coping strategy, it's important to match it to the emotional energy that you have. High-energy emotions like anger and anxiety often respond well to activities that involve noteworthy exertion, whether that is aerobic effort, strength, endurance, or some combination. The point is to discharge excess energy, both physically and emotionally. Easy choices for this include working out, bicycling, jogging, power-walking, dancing, heavy household or yard work of any kind, or anything else that makes you work hard toward a constructive end.

If you're experiencing a low-energy emotion like sadness, depression, grief, or discouragement, physical activity is still highly useful, but the choices will be different. Here, you'll probably be better served by strolling, stretching, household tasks that are not strenuous, or perhaps some light errands. You *don't* want to tire yourself out if you're already in a low-energy state; pushing too hard can make you feel worse rather than better. The goal is to use your time and limited energy in ways that gently create some positive results in your life, helping you to feel better and more able as you do.

You can adapt various activities to the required energy level simply by changing how intensely you do them. If you have a high-energy emotion to discharge and the only activity available to you is walking, for example, you can stomp around your neighborhood with more than enough vigor to get the job done. On the other hand, if you're having a low-energy day but have to do something moderately strenuous like heavy housework, just do it slowly. Most of your options needn't be pigeonholed as either high-energy or low-energy; varying the intensity gives most of them some utility toward either end of the spectrum.

A final note about coping via physical activity is that we are all unique. The suggestions above will be useful for many people, but may not fit for you. Some people prefer to deal with high-energy emotions by moderating them—via yoga or meditation, for example—rather than working them off. Some people with low-energy emotions may find that a demanding activity effectively snaps them out of it, at least sometimes. The only way you'll know for sure is to experiment with different options to find out what works best for you.

Bad feelings get a lot less intimidating when you know you have effective ways to deal with them. You've probably turned to food for relief of those feelings many, many times, hoping it would help but finding additional disappointment instead. The great thing about physical activity is that it actually *does* help.

Have Some Personal Interests

As mentioned previously, you'll have a more interesting and enjoyable life if you have a hobby or two, in addition to having more of a buffer against the stresses of life as they arise.

A good hobby gives you something to enjoy, something to look forward to, and something to plan around because you find it important enough to prioritize it. In a world where we are often defined in reference to others—you are someone's child; you may be someone's spouse, someone's employee, someone's boss, etc.—a hobby allows you to experience yourself in your own skin, having your own experience, for your own sake. In a culture that is increasingly fast-paced and fragmented, a hobby creates an oasis of personal peace and focus that can be found in few other ways. It allows you to experience moments when time stands still as you immerse yourself fully in what you are doing.

You can enjoy *all* of these benefits from an act as simple as taking quiet time for yourself to read something purely for pleasure. It's so easy and costs so little, yet has come to feel like the ultimate luxury for many who have trouble finding time in their lives to slow down for a bit and just *be*.

Should you have the ability to develop an activity-based hobby, you'll find that time spent at it allows you to change things up. You get to focus your energy differently, use different skills, overcome different challenges, and maybe even enjoy a change in scenery, depending on what you're doing.

If you are someone who tends to experience self-doubt, your hobby can be a source of confidence that subtly spills over into other aspects of your life.

If your hobby involves interaction with others, it can broaden your social network and be a source of new friends, thus contributing to two important parts of your life rather than just one.

Likewise, if your hobby happens to involve potentially marketable skills, it can even open up additional opportunities for the employment part of your life.

If you're the creative type, you may find some form of visual art to be an enjoyable way to spend time. You may also discover it to be a powerful means of self-expression, especially if you're not as comfortable as you'd like to be with verbal communication. Artistic work communicates on many levels; you may find that the more you practice it, the better you get at finding the words to communicate verbally as well.

Finally, a hobby can be a source of refuge during painful times. It gives you a familiar emotional space where you can do familiar things, experiencing comforting routines that assure you of some continuity in life even as you deal with challenges and change.

For all of these reasons, hobbies are wonderful assets and sources of reward for your emotional brain. Having one won't eliminate your food urges, but it will help.

Distractions of the Enjoyable, Constructive, and Productive Kind

If bad things are happening in your inner world, you can actually offset them a bit by making some good things happen in your outer world.

One way to do that is to take advantage of enjoyable activities that you usually miss out on because you lack the time. If you're having a bad enough day, you're probably wasting the time anyway.

Why not pull out that novel you've wanted to read or visit that beautiful park you've been eyeing from afar? Any *it-would-just-be-nice* kind of thing will do. With any luck, you'll get some actual enjoyment out of your choice but even if you don't, you will have spent the time in a positive way rather than in a way that makes things worse.

Another way to manage one of these difficult times is to choose to do something that will improve the quality of your outer world, whether or not you happen to enjoy the process as you do it.

You can accomplish this with the simplest of acts, like putting on some enjoyable music and washing that pile of dishes in the kitchen that's been depressing you. You could try changing the sheets on your bed (even if they don't absolutely need it yet) so that if nothing else, the bed will feel extra comfy tonight. You might like how it feels to straighten up one limited bit of clutter in an important room so that you can feel better when you spend time there.

Look for little things you can do that will make your space feel more comfortable and inviting for you. Actions like these will probably help you today, but even if they don't, you'll have changed your immediate space in ways that lift you up more than they pull you down. It'll be easier to feel better sooner, even if it doesn't happen today, and you might also feel a little better about yourself for choosing to do something positive even though it took some effort.

An alternative approach that may surprise you is to make a point of knocking off a bunch of chores, tasks, and errands that you actively dislike, but which are necessary nonetheless. Since you're already having a bad day, you won't make it worse by taking care of needed business that you don't happen to enjoy. You'll get things done that will no longer be hanging over you, which will give you a nice feeling of liberation from the unwanted. You'll spend the time productively, which will remind you that you have the power to make things better for yourself. Your life will be measurably better as a result of your efforts, which will help you to climb out of the bad mood more easily.

The important thing to remember about strategies like these is that when you use them, you are keeping your way of life intact during a time when you might feel more like just letting it crumble for a while.

The problem with letting it crumble at all is that your way of life, itself, then becomes more depressing. If the way you live becomes a disorganized mess that would depress anyone, your path to feeling better is much more challenging—doable, but harder. Why let it be harder than it has to be? No matter how bad you feel, keep going through the motions of keeping your life operational.

Future You will thank you for it.

Brighten Someone Else's Day

You've probably heard of the notion of performing random acts of kindness, and you may have assumed this to be about simple altruism: one person doing something for another without expectation of personal gain. As inspiring as that is, it's rarely possible to perform a truly altruistic act, because—*who knew??*—the emotional brain is wired to like doing nice things for other people.[2]

If you've ever been generous or kind in some way just because you felt like it and then noticed some nice, warm feelings of your own afterwards, that was your emotional brain registering a potent internal reward. Ask someone who volunteers about why they do it, and they'll most often answer that it's because they find it personally rewarding—it *feels* good.

If you're having a bad day, extending kindness toward someone else will do several important things for *you*. It will show you that you are capable of doing something positive even when you're not in a good emotional place, which reminds you that you have value in the world even when you don't feel like you do. It will remind you of the power we all have, to be an uplifting presence to another human being at any time. It will shift your attention away from being stuck and toward being effective, thus helping you to regain personal traction. Finally, it will have a healing effect directly at the source of your own suffering: your emotional brain.

For all of these reasons, doing for others is a remarkably effective way to lift your own spirits. What's amazing is how little effort it takes to generate benefits of such magnitude.

The simplest acts make a difference that can be felt and enjoyed by both you and the person with whom you share the moment. Make an extra effort to hold a door for someone, make space for another driver to merge into heavy traffic, or give away your place in line at a busy store. Your action may simply brighten a moment in someone else's life, or it may so alter the course of their day that they tell their family all about it when they get home that night. You'll never know how much of a difference you made, but you'll know that you made one.

Compliments are an easy way to do for others. Let someone know that their warm demeanor brightens your day, you admire how well they parent their kids, or that their particular talents and dependability make your life easier.

Just share whatever it is that you notice and appreciate, because they probably don't hear it much. When you interact with someone who works with the public all day, for example, you can show them that you *see* them when you acknowledge how patient and helpful they are even though it must be frustrating for them at times.

Feeling too uncomfortable to interact much? Just make eye contact with others when you can, and smile. It is a simple act with the power to acknowledge the presence and humanity of the other person. It offers friendliness, openness, and warmth, even if no words are ever spoken. For just a moment, it creates a fleeting human connection which is likely to be beneficial in some barely conscious way to each party. You get a tiny little lift, and so do they.

If you have trouble working up a smile for a stranger or worry that you'll come across as fake if you try, a thought experiment might help. It commonly happens that when someone has an accident or a medical crisis in public, they are assisted with great compassion and urgency by total strangers. After the event, those who needed the help and those who provided it end up feeling a warm personal bond.

So here's your thought experiment: You're walking along in a public place, just about to cross paths with a stranger you will probably never see again. Maybe you'd rather not smile because you feel bad anyway and would prefer to stay in your own little personal cocoon.

Consider how rapidly your heart would open if that person had a crisis in front of you (took a bad fall, got hit by a car, dropped with a heart attack) and you could see a way to help. Consider how rapidly your heart would open if *you* had a crisis in front of them and realized that they were there for you in your moment of need.

Either way, the emotional distance would vanish in an instant. When you look at that stranger for the second or two that your eyes will meet, try smiling as you think, "Thank you for the friend you would instantly be if my life depended on it." The smile you give as you have that thought will be a warm one that you both enjoy, and which lifts both your days just a bit.

You needn't do this with every person you encounter, though you certainly can if you want to. If you have low emotional energy, it can be effective to set a goal for yourself, like five connect-with-another-human-being smiles in a day, or whatever number suits you. You can get them all done early in the day if you want more of the emotional boost sooner, or you can spread them throughout the day if you worry about using up too much energy all at once. The right way to do it is whatever way works the best for you.

Doing for others—however big or small your act may be—reminds you of how simple it is to get more positive energy flowing in your own life at any time. No matter how far down you are, you *always* have the power to brighten the life of someone else, and you'll take one step back toward feeling better each time you do.

Meditation, Relaxation, and Prayer

It has been my observation that many more people are willing to make the time for prayer than for meditation or relaxation, and that most people would benefit from doing any of the three a lot more often. Most people feel that they lack the time; it's a busy, hectic life and there are just so many other things that have to be done.

Meditation, relaxation, and prayer are different practices which yield very similar benefits. They each provide a welcome respite from the pressures of the moment. Each calms the physical reactions associated with stress while quieting the mind. Each connects you to that which makes you more peaceful, strong, and centered. You emerge from each more refreshed and clear, able to manage your life more positively and effectively.

This remarkable transformation is always available to you, provided you take the time for the practices that make it possible. Because the relevant neural pathways get stronger each time you use them, regular practice means that the beneficial results will come to you more quickly and easily over time—the more you practice, the better it gets.

Journaling

Journaling isn't the tool of choice for everyone, but offers an impressive array of benefits for those who do it.

It's particularly good for getting you moving again when you're feeling emotionally stuck. Distressed people tend to ruminate on their problems, constantly replaying the same thoughts over and over again in their heads, gaining neither clarity nor solutions in the process. There is something about the act of getting thoughts like that into print that often breaks the cycle, allowing them to progress rather than continuing to spin in place.

When that happens, you are likely to gain a better understanding of what is going on inside of you. This is important because when all you know about your emotional state is that you don't like it, there's no way to know how to make it better. Swirling storms of unnamed feelings all create the same end result: generic pain in search of generic relief. This is the perfect setup for turning to food, a generic solution that also happens to be readily available.

The treachery of seeking emotional relief through food is that it improves nothing, while creating secondary problems that will cause you to need even more relief in the future. If you can start pinning down what the feelings actually are, you can begin to break this cycle.

When you start pouring out your thoughts and feelings in writing, generic pain starts to reveal its true components: frustration, anxiety, helplessness, hopelessness, anger, disappointment, grief, betrayal, sadness, uncertainty, impatience, depression, or being overwhelmed. These aren't all of the possibilities, but it gives you an idea of the specificity that lies just below the surface when you are feeling emotionally out of sorts.

Once you've identified the real feelings in question, you're in a position to perform effective emotional first aid for yourself. You can choose from strategies like those in this chapter, customizing your efforts to the feelings that you're having.

High-energy feelings might be best served through physical activity and staying productively busy, while low-energy feelings might respond well to getting more support from others or seeking comfort in a familiar hobby, for example. You can choose strategies that actually help you feel better, rather than turning to food which offers nothing but temporary distraction and numbness.

Whatever the feelings are, maximizing your self-care activities is always a good idea; when you need a generic strategy, that's the one that will actually help. What's the simplest way to increase your self-care in a moment of emotional distress? Go for a walk. It helps quickly, and it's nearly as available as food. I have yet to hear of anyone, anywhere who hasn't found this helpful during a bad time (provided they had a safe place in which to do it). Walking may not solve the immediate problem, but it will help you to get your head together a bit while also giving you some safe distance from food at a time when you're vulnerable. It's an easy win at a time when you need one.

Journaling often makes it easier to identify aspects of your life that may be fueling your troubled feelings, such as a strained relationship, work-related stress, or financial worries. Once you've identified the source of your unrest, you can begin problem-solving and developing a plan of action.

Your first and most important task is to begin assessing whether your own perspective might be adding to your distress. Is it possible that you've taken something too personally? Are you making assumptions based on incomplete information? Could you be assuming the worst and discounting information that would help you to see things in a more favorable light?

As it turns out, we add to our own misery in these and other creative ways when we are distressed; a particularly good book on the subject is *Feeling Good: The New Mood Therapy*.[3] It has had remarkable staying power in the crowded world of self-help literature for years because what it teaches is so useful. It is an excellent resource for learning how to examine your thinking and discover the ways in which you inadvertently increase your own distress.

Through guided written exercises, you can develop effective strategies for more objective, empowering styles of thought, literally calming your emotional brain and strengthening the role of your cortex. The level of change that is possible is amazing, and it's a simple matter of training and practice. The book is designed to be used for self-help, but the material is well known in the therapy world; if you try it on your own and get stuck, most therapists can help you work out the kinks so that you'll be back on track in short order.

Assessing your own thinking is a task of primary importance because it is not your life situation, but the way you look at it, that has the strongest impact on how you feel and how effective you will ultimately be. It is therefore vital to assure that your perception is as fact-based as possible so that you can make the best use of whatever reality you have. A balanced perspective positions you to develop targeted solutions to clearly defined problems rather than continuing to suffer endlessly in some generalized way that you don't fully understand. Journaling is a highly effective way in which to achieve that perspective.

Journaling is not something you need to do every day—or even on a regular basis—unless you want to. The time to journal is when you have something to say, something to explore, or something to try to sort out. Even if journaling brings no further clarity at all, it's still likely to give you some relief simply because you've off-loaded some painful energy. Better that than to try masking your feelings with food.

The question clients most often ask about journaling is, "How do I start?" The answer is that you simply start writing whatever you're thinking, and just see where it takes you. It might start out like this:

> *Well, okay. Here I am. Writing is supposed to help, but I don't know what to write and I'm not very good at it anyway. I hate that I even have to think about doing something like this. It isn't bad enough that I have to feel crappy in the first place, let alone that I have to take time to sit down and write about it!*
>
> *It's just so discouraging. I feel like I bang my head against the wall every day and nothing ever gets better …*

What you see in the example above is fairly typical, in that it usually doesn't take long to shift from aimlessly fumbling around to beginning to articulate some feelings that can be explored further. Once that begins, you're on your way to figuring out how you can start making things better for yourself.

It's Non-Food Strategies That Make Your Life Better
All of the strategies described in this chapter provide excellent support for your emotional brain and quality care for your body.

They provide considerable leverage in containing the urge to overeat, while protecting and improving your quality of life.

They help to restore your perspective when you need it the most, positioning you to evaluate your challenges more accurately and address them more effectively. This in turn helps you to create and maintain a far more satisfying life in which food naturally becomes less important.

They provide numerous ways to strengthen your self-confidence along with building authentic hope for the future. They keep you attuned to the power you always have—and the wide variety of ways in which you can use it—to turn your life for the better and keep it moving in that direction.

Strategies like these are the only way out of the emotional unrest that drives you toward food. Turning to food for emotional reasons, on the other hand, guarantees that the torment will never end.

Chapter 25
Taking Care of Yourself When You Least Feel Like It

When the chips are down, many people start letting go of the practices that make their lives feel good and work well. They start eating lower-quality food that has a great flavor hit while lacking nutritional substance. They start spending more time eating and less time on other, more life-affirming personal interests that would take more commitment. They become more sedentary, telling themselves that they lack the time and energy right now for more active pursuits. With each choice of this type, a little more life quality is allowed to slip away and the emotional hole gets a little deeper.

I have long observed that most of the people who come to me for help with overeating also have a history of recurrent depression. When I say "most," I mean close to 90%—the correlation is incredibly strong.

The choices you're attracted to during your low times—declining physical activity and lots of junky food—are poor building blocks for a quality life in any event, but they also increase systemic inflammation. This increases your risk for many medical problems, including depression itself.[1]

So, in yet another cruel irony, the choices you feel most attracted to in your depression are the choices that will intensify it rather than providing relief. You want to feel better, but you feel drawn to the choices that will make you feel worse.

Depression is far more than just a bad feeling. Depression, in the medical sense, refers to suppressed functioning of the nervous system. Because your nervous system is intertwined with every other system in your body, the symptoms of depression are quite varied.

In addition to a depressed mood, you may experience other symptoms like low energy, loss of motivation, loss of enjoyment, isolating yourself from supportive others, self-critical thoughts, mental fogginess, eating too much or too little, sleeping too much or too little, crying more of the time, feeling anxious, feeling generally slowed, and feeling pessimistic about your prospects for being okay again.

Depressive episodes don't have to involve every single one of these symptoms, though it can happen. Having *any* of them is a sign that you need to step up your self-care immediately and start paying close attention to whether or not you are improving over time, because you might be able to keep depression from settling in if you work at it intentionally. The challenge is that you need to tackle it aggressively at just the time when you're beginning to feel apathetic and unmotivated.

Sometimes though, depression will overtake you despite your best efforts, dragging on or getting worse no matter what you do. If you've done everything you can and you're still not okay, getting some help will get you back to feeling like yourself a lot sooner than if you keep waiting it out.

Counseling is a good place to start; a licensed psychotherapist can provide valuable support and help with coping skills, along with an assessment of whether medication should be considered. Medication may or may not be suggested, but if it is, your therapist can coordinate with your family doctor or any psychiatric professional so that you can get all the help you need.

Deeply depressed people sometimes come to believe that the emotional pain will never end and that death is the only way out. Many have had some version of this thought: *I'd never do anything to hurt myself, but if I died in my sleep tonight, that would be okay.* Some become so desperate for the pain to stop that they contemplate suicide; tragically, some follow through.

I have spoken to many depressed people at times when they were preoccupied with death, but I recall no one who—when they really thought about it—actually wanted to die. What they all wanted was simply for the pain to stop. Death only looked attractive because their thinking had become so narrowed by their depression that they couldn't imagine any other solutions.

It is very important, should you ever find yourself thinking this way, to remember that *this is a symptom of depression* rather than a sign that life is actually no longer worth living. If that's the way you're feeling, it means you've got a medical issue that is interfering with your ability to think and feel like yourself. It's time to get some help. Now.

Because depressive episodes can sometimes be nipped in the bud, it's important to know what to watch for in order to catch them early. Consider how you live, think, and behave when life is good and you're at your best, then try to notice the earliest possible stages of beginning to behave in ways that are "not like you" in your ideal state.

If you're usually quite active and the couch has seemed more inviting in recent days, look carefully at what that might mean. Maybe you've exerted yourself quite a bit lately and some rest makes perfect sense. Maybe you're experiencing fatigue associated with some brewing medical issue that should be addressed.

Or maybe you just don't feel like doing much of anything; nothing seems all that important or interesting. That should be a red flag, because if you normally like to be active and are feeling a loss of interest, that's not like you and that means something.

If it's the beginning of a depressive slide, push yourself while you still can and keep moving. It *will* help, and you *will* be glad that you did. If the depression is getting enough of a grip that it's difficult to maintain your normal level of exertion, then just do what you can. The important thing is that you do not succumb to the siren song of the couch (or your bed)—there is nothing good there for you.

Likewise, if you normally eat well but start feeling like it's too much bother, that's a sign. Did you used to have take-out as an occasional fun change of pace, but now find that it's something you do a few times a week? Have you been skimping on breakfast when you used to consider it important to have a good one every day? Have you been using snack machines at times when you previously would have planned and prepared more nutritional snacks to bring with you?

If you find that you've wandered from the patterns that you enjoy when you're at your best, it means you're not fully okay. Now is the time to purposefully correct your course, before these changes steal more of your energy than they already have. If you want to start feeling better, you need to start eating better immediately.

If you normally connect with friends and family on a regular basis but don't find that as appealing lately, it may be cause for concern. Is there a practical reason for it that you can understand, or is it that you just don't feel the interest? Do you find yourself thinking that you don't have much to offer your loved ones anyway, and that they probably have better ways to spend their time? Do you feel like you just don't have anything to say to anyone? If so, that's a warning that depression could be lurking. Reach out to your loved ones even though you don't feel like it. It will help.

Is there something you've long enjoyed doing that has inexplicably lost its appeal to you? It may be an activity or hobby that has brightened your life for years; people who know you may even think of it as a core part of who you are. If you don't care for it any more, you need to take a closer look at why. Perhaps this activity fit in your life for a long time and now you're just growing into new interests and directions; if so, that's a healthy process in which you're simply pruning away that which no longer adds value.

If, however, you've cooled on this past interest of yours and are not embracing anything new to take its place, that means you're in a state of contraction rather than change, which is a hallmark sign of depression.

It would be a good idea to keep going through the motions of your activity for now even though you lack the interest. It is simply better depression management to stay engaged in something—however half-heartedly—than to allow your life to shrink. You will find that as the depression lifts, your motivation will return.

Then you'll be in a better position to determine whether it's time for change and if so, what new things you'd like to try. Until then, the smart move is to keep your life moving in the ways that you know how, even though you don't feel like it.

Your own thoughts may be your biggest obstacle to staving off a budding depression, so beware of any inner rationalizations about how you haven't changed that much yet or how it hasn't been going on for very long.

If you're not behaving like yourself, something's up—you may be seeing the early signs of an emotional descent. Your best chances at turning it around are early on rather than once it's well under way, so it pays to be proactive.

Plan A then, is to stay out of the hole in the first place if you can. When you first notice some slippage in your habits, you still have some energy reserves because it hasn't gotten too bad yet. This is the time to start fighting hard for yourself.

Don't lie back, give up, and tell yourself how tired you are, hoping things will feel better soon. It will be difficult, but it's essential that you get to work doing those things that reliably make your life better, and that you maintain the effort even if it doesn't seem to be producing results right away. You have some chance of reversing the depression but even if you can't do that, you might still be able to minimize how bad it gets.

If depression settles in anyway, Plan B is to focus on maintaining your self-care the best you can while you reach out for some help. No matter how you feel, keep working the problem to the best of your ability—if you go down fighting, you probably won't go down quite as far.

It's actually possible to have symptoms of depression and *not* be clinically depressed, provided you don't have them for very long. Anyone might temporarily have symptoms of this type in response to a personal hardship, setback, or loss, but then start the slow process of recovering within a matter of days.

If you're having an understandably painful reaction to something that has gone wrong in your life, it's important to keep taking the best care of yourself that you can as you go through it, even though you don't feel like it. If you're not seeing the beginning of any recovery process within a couple of weeks and are having trouble keeping up with the basic requirements of your life, then you need to consider the possibility of depression.

If you're like most people, you'll decide to wait longer than that, hoping that you'll start to come around on your own. If you are able to see incremental progress over time as your suffering slowly decreases, you're probably in a healthy process of adjustment that is just going to take some time. Getting extra support at this point isn't strictly necessary, though it will probably ease your suffering if you do.

If you're continuing to remain stuck in the same emotional place week after week, however, that means there's no end in sight—you're definitely better off seeking help rather than continuing to wait.

If you're depressed and it doesn't seem to be getting better, whether you can explain what caused it or not, please remember this: Depression is a medical condition and effective treatment is available. Life is too short to suffer with it when you don't have to.

Chapter 26

Thinking More Effectively About Food

Whether or not you realize it, you talk to yourself in your thoughts a great deal of the time, giving internal voice to how you see yourself and everything in your world. The tone and language of that self-talk has an enormous impact on your perception and on how well you navigate the challenges in your life, so it pays to assure that you are using it as well as possible.

When it comes to self-care in general and food in particular, *should* may be the word we use the most. We create mental lists of the good choices we should be making, then berate ourselves for not following through. We think of all the bad things we shouldn't be doing—but are doing anyway—and berate ourselves for those, too. This is the approach most of us have used for decades now, during which time the vast majority of us have become steadily heavier and sicker.

Terms like *should, shouldn't, good,* and *bad* are loaded terms in that they often inspire a negative reaction in the emotional brain. Nobody likes to be told what they should or shouldn't do, and we don't like hearing it from our own internal voice any more than we like hearing it from the people around us.

It's important to understand that your internal self-talk has just as much power as anything others can ever say to you. In fact, your self-talk is *more* powerful simply because it is ever-present.

Imagine someone having constant access to you, following you around and whispering in your ear through every waking moment of every day, no matter what you are doing (let's say that you've somehow accepted this and are not horrified by the idea of someone shadowing you at all times).

This could be okay if the person is trustworthy, supportive, and able to offer good ideas when you need them. But what if that person is judgmental, demanding, and critical, bombarding you with withering condemnations and ordering you around all day?

No one has the access to do that to us, thank goodness, but our own self-talk *is* that constant and inescapable. We need to be aware of it and to assure that we are using it to our best advantage rather than in ways that undermine the life we want the most.

When you tell yourself that you should be eating better and exercising more, the message welling up from your emotional brain may be, *But I don't want to and you can't make me.* When you tell yourself that soda is a bad choice and that you shouldn't drink it, the emotional brain replies, *Oh yeah? Watch this,* as you reach for the bottle.

Directive self-talk—*you should do this, you shouldn't do that*—sometimes works, but is high-risk as a primary strategy simply because it so often ends up goading the emotional brain into a rebellious power grab instead. It is the job of the cortex to craft a stream of self-talk that keeps the emotional brain open to helpful suggestion rather than triggering it into resistance.

Language Substitutions That Help

You can dramatically improve the effectiveness of your self-talk merely by getting rid of language that provokes emotional pushback. It helps if you focus instead on neutral, descriptive information that helps you to evaluate your options more objectively.

For example, many people categorize food as either *good for you* or *bad for you.* Good and bad are value judgments, not descriptions, which is why they trigger an emotional reaction.

Instead of *good for you,* think about the facts associated with the food we describe that way. Food of this type makes your body stronger, more resistant to disease, and able to repair itself more effectively when necessary. When your diet consists mostly of this kind of food, you feel better, both physically and emotionally. You also have more options for enjoying yourself since you have greater physical vitality.

Likewise, think about the facts associated with the food we commonly refer to as *bad for you.* Such food has great entertainment value, but fails to provide the nutrients that your body needs in order to be strong and function well. It often contains substances that contribute to a variety of disease processes. Eating a lot of it results in both physical and emotional decline over time. Options for enjoying life are reduced due to susceptibility to depression and dwindling physical ability. Eating a lot of this food makes you old before your time.

Think about how you react to the concepts of *good for you* and *bad for you*, and notice the difference in how you feel when you read the more objective descriptions above. You may feel less inclined toward rebellion when you look at the simple facts. No value judgments, no *shoulds* or *shouldn'ts* ... just facts.

You'll probably still want some foods of nominal nutritional value in your life simply because you enjoy them so much, but at least you'll be relieved of the extra burden of craving the forbidden. Food of this nature is not forbidden. It just comes with a list of ugly side effects that you need to take into account as you decide what role to allow it in your life.

Focusing attentively on the facts will dramatically reduce the emotional pull associated with trigger foods. If you're lucky, sometimes the facts alone will be enough for you to feel okay about walking away. At the very least, they will help you to think more clearly as you decide what to do, perhaps choosing a less damaging path than you otherwise would have. Facts are your friends—they help tremendously in making those decisions that work out well both in the moment and long afterward.

Often though, we don't have the time or patience to think through all of that. We default to summary labels like *good* and *bad* because they're easy. Since the emotional brain likes quick-and-easy labels and is going to continue using them anyway, the solution is to come up with better ones.

The best language to use is that which feels natural, helpful, and inviting to you. One possibility is to categorize various edibles simply as either food or not-food. Food refers to nontoxic plants and animals and minimally processed products made from them, the consumption of which contributes to physical health. Not-food refers to manufactured ingredients and products that are edible but which are not useful in supporting health, and which have the potential to trigger overeating.[1]

The latter might also be thought of as treat foods, in recognition of the fact that they are indeed enjoyable even if they have nothing else to offer. When considering how much space in your life to allot to such products, it is important to realize that eating them is about fun, not food, and that your body still needs food in any event. Considering these decisions based on facts rather than judgments will position you to make choices that serve you better, meeting your needs for both enjoyment and good health.

If the food/not-food approach doesn't work for you, here are some questions to consider asking yourself about each of the edibles in your life, which may help you to discover the method of labeling that is easiest and most effective for you:

- Is it more likely to help you or to hurt you?

- Does it primarily make you stronger or weaker?

- Is it most likely to result in your feeling better about yourself, or worse?

- Does it support your goals or does it undermine them?

- Does it mostly move you forward or pull you backward?

- Does it bring you closer to the life you most want or take you further from it?

Any of these questions or others like them will help you to evaluate your options more effectively. The key is to find a way to think about food that is accurate and personally meaningful, which enables you to make calmer and more controlled decisions about what, when, how, and why you eat.

How to Stop Picking Fights with Your Emotional Brain

Once you've figured out a more useful way to label your options, it's a good idea to look for other aspects of your self-talk that might trigger an unwanted reaction in your emotional brain.

It always concerns me a little when I hear someone talk about what they *allow* themselves, e.g., "I allow myself a snack every evening." It's not the snack that gives me pause—it's the possibility that the concept of *allowing* might stir up trouble in the emotional brain. I don't wish to discourage you if you have made effective use of this concept and find that it keeps you happily and successfully on track year after year; if it works that way for you, keep right on using it.

The problem is that there are many people for whom it does *not* work, though they often keep trying it anyway. In those cases, there are two ways in which it is most likely to go wrong. First, if you *allow* a behavior at some times, that implies the behavior is *not allowed* at other times. This calls up those *good/bad* and *should/shouldn't* dichotomies that prove so provocative to the emotional brain.

The second way that *allowing* can go wrong is when it implies a situation of ongoing deprivation from which an occasional reprieve is granted. The emotional brain will respond to this in the only way that makes sense: a relentless desire to escape.

In either case, it is not a question of whether your efforts will eventually fall apart, because they assuredly will. It's only a matter of when.

A related concept is that of the "cheat day" or "cheat meal" that many of my clients have mentioned. The idea is that if you're *good* for enough of the time, you can *cheat* on a limited basis and still have things work out okay. Unfortunately, I most often hear of "cheat" meals or days that easily undo all the progress made in the remainder of the week, as the emotional brain scrambles to maximize the time-limited free pass while it lasts.

Rather than the emotional mess created by *good, bad, should, shouldn't, allowing, not allowing, cheating,* and all similar modes of thought, I suggest that you simply focus instead on questions like these:

- What *works* for you? What makes you stronger, more focused, and more successful with your food and other self-care decisions? Not just for days or weeks at a time, but for the long haul, without causing you annoyance or disappointment? Anything you can identify—no matter how small—will be an important piece of the successful system you eventually design. The more such little pieces you can identify, the better.

- What do you find genuinely helpful? What makes it easier for you to pursue the kinds of choices you'd really like to be making more of the time?

- Which patterns, strategies, and choices help you to feel the best by the end of each day?

If you can't come up with many answers yet, just keep the questions in mind as you go forward. Stay on the lookout for answers you may have missed simply because you weren't looking for them until now. You will find that a system based on this kind of thinking is one that makes it easier to sidestep the actions you'd later regret, favor the actions that will make you the happiest, and feel good about the process throughout.

To help you get going, here are some generic answers to the questions above, based on statements I've heard from numerous clients:

- <u>What works for you?</u> *Having an easy breakfast every day. Having good leftovers ready for easy lunches. Knowing ahead of time which part of my day will be best for an exercise break. Cooking in batches so I don't have to cook as often. Planning a fun snack to look forward to so that I can just focus on nutritious food the rest of the day, assuring that the portion size of the snack will not be big enough to interfere with my goals.*

- <u>What do you find genuinely helpful?</u> *Keeping a lot of quality food on hand so I always have some easy choices. Keeping trigger foods out of my home. Eating out a lot less than I used to, because it's easier to control myself at home than it is in most restaurants. Making plans with friends that are about doing something together other than just sharing a meal. Keeping myself busy during those times of the day when I'm most likely to want to focus too much on food.*

- <u>Which patterns, strategies, and choices help you to feel the best by the end of each day?</u> *Making sure that I do something for exercise almost every day, because when I start skipping it more, I usually drop it soon after. Thinking about who I want to be and the life I want to have, and whether or not the food choices that tempt me fit into that. Being aware of which foods make me lose control and staying away from them as much as I can. Just trying my best and learning what I can from the times that go wrong so I can be stronger as a result.*

There's one more common style of thinking about self-care choices that merits mention, and that is the establishment of personal *rules*, often identified by that name. The one I hear mentioned most often is, "I have a rule that I never eat after (a certain hour of the evening)." This thinking style can be either damaging or helpful, depending entirely on how you define *rules*.

If you think of rules as dictates that must be obeyed, your emotional brain is likely to resist at some point. If so, you'll probably have thoughts along these lines: *Rules were made to be broken ... All rules have exceptions ... Rule? What rule? ... I don't care—I'm eating it anyway.* If your self-care-related rules feel like edicts to you, they are unlikely to be helpful in the long run.

On the other hand, if you think of rules as guidelines that make your life better, they can be an excellent strategy. For comparison, consider the rules we usually follow when we drive. We drive at the speed limit or not too much above it. We signal turns before making them. We yield when making a turn across opposing traffic. We turn our headlights on when it gets dark. We slow down in bad weather. We stop at red lights, no matter how rushed we feel.

There are many, many rules that we submit to when we drive; we usually do so without resentment because to drive without them would be suicide. These limitations have the ironic effect of creating immense freedom of movement; they don't oppress us—they keep us safe. If you have rules related to food and self-care that feel *that* way to you, do carry on. Such rules create a safe structure within which you can relax and enjoy your food more fully.

A common rule that serves many of us well, for example, is to eat only while sitting down (not including vehicles). It's a simple way to increase your awareness of when and what you're eating—as long as you're paying enough attention to make the choice. Rules like this do nothing to restrict your eating, but they do help you to pay attention and choose more carefully. They're a big help, actually.

If you like the idea of beneficial rules but are still put off by the word *rule*, then just don't use it. You can simply craft a number of statements about what you do and don't do, all chosen based on how they improve your quality of life with food; it ends up being a simple description of what you do and how you live.

If naming it makes it easier to think and talk about, consider a neutral term like *system*—used occasionally in this text—to describe that set of practices you are developing in order to create the life, health, and relationship with food that you want. Whatever you call it (if anything), how you *feel* about it is ultimately the best predictor of how well it will serve you.

Common Thought Traps

One of the interesting elements of any addiction is that those who share it come to think in some similar and predictable ways. Overeating is no exception, so I'll offer a few of the most common thoughts here (in the gray clouds below), along with examples of how they can be countered. And they really *need* to be countered because they have a lot to do with why you've remained stuck for so long. You will remain stuck—or at least struggling a lot harder with change than you have to—if you don't challenge thoughts like these.

The suggestions you'll see here are not the only possible countermeasures. They are simply ideas for you to consider so that you can adopt them if you like them, or improve upon them if you can.

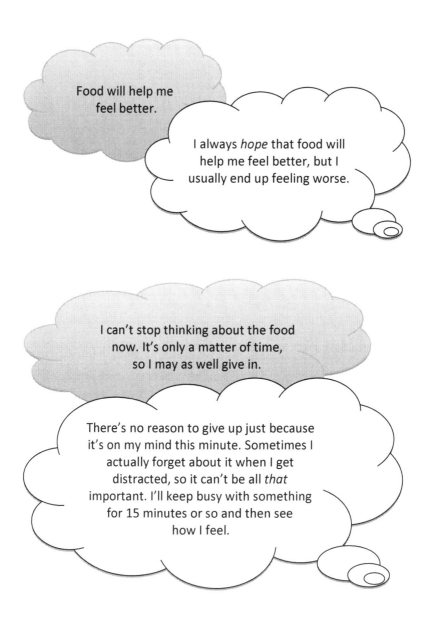

It's a special occasion! Lots of fun food is just part of celebrating!

It's just food. I can get any of it at any time if I really want to. There's nothing here I need to hurt myself over. There's nothing here that I will be happy to have overeaten. The last time I overate under these circumstances, I felt terrible about it afterwards.

I've been good today, so I can have an extra treat!

I've already planned for treats that I know will work for me. If I eat more than that, I'll just end up regretting it.

I messed up the day already anyway, so what difference does it make?

I'll have less of a mess to recover from if I stop the damage now. I can keep this from getting worse, and I'll be glad that I did.

I don't care—I just want it!

I *will* care later. I'll end up really wishing I hadn't done it, because that's the way this always turns out. I can't remember ever doing this and feeling happy about it afterward.

I'll make up for this by eating less and exercising more tomorrow.

It's hard on me to bounce between extremes like that. I feel better when I just stay closer to the middle most of the time.

I don't get to have this special food very often, so I need to take advantage of it while I can.

I can request it, buy it, or make it any time if I want it badly enough. There's no need to get excited about it just because it's sitting here right now.

It's been a rough day. I deserve a reward.

I deserve a reward that doesn't make me feel bad later. Feeling stuffed and ashamed is not rewarding.

Hey, food is just part of enjoying life to the fullest!

Yes, but not the way I've been doing it. I don't enjoy hating myself afterwards.

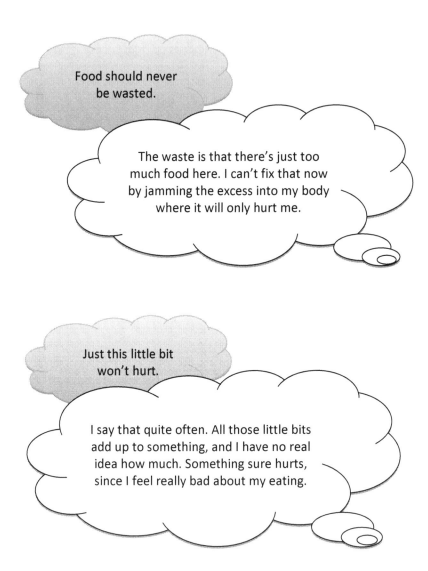

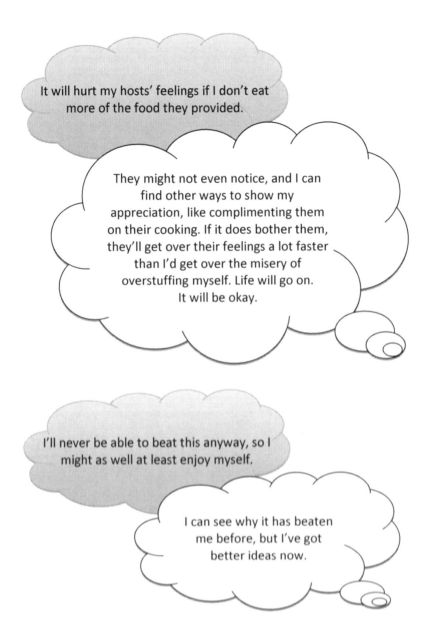

As you can see, the way you talk to yourself about your options makes all the difference in the choices you ultimately make. The key is to stay focused on the life you really want and the facts that keep you on track in creating it. The more you practice intentionally thinking in this manner, the more easily it will come to you over time.

Chapter 27
Planning for Long-Term Success

You understand by now that your emotional brain is primed to react quickly and intensely to food triggers, and that this is not likely to change much over the remainder of your life. However, our society still promotes the myth that control with food is just a matter of willpower. As a result, millions of us have spent years mistakenly condemning ourselves for lack of self-discipline when the real problem is that we've been living in an environment that causes most people to struggle with food.

Willpower is indeed a powerful engine for success ... in those life endeavors that don't involve repeatedly going up against a primal survival imperative like the drive to acquire food. History doesn't even suggest that it *should* work, given that most of humanity has lived in conditions of food scarcity where willpower was simply unnecessary. It's only in recent times that we've unwittingly conducted the experiment of exposing large populations to easy-access, hyperpalatable food, and the results are in. Willpower is not the answer.

We all have some capacity for willpower, of course, but few have it at the levels required to remain in control of their eating in such a triggering environment. The structure and function of the brain just don't support it. Since willpower can't reliably contain the urge to overeat in these conditions, the best defense is to minimize how often and how intensely we are confronted with the urge.

The Importance of Planning

The theme that emerges most consistently from my clinical work with overeaters is the need for more planning with food. Spontaneous food decisions need to be minimized because they are almost always made by the emotional brain, typically when it's already unbalanced due to hunger, stress, distraction, or fatigue. The emotional brain is bad at figuring out food in the modern world to begin with, but it's even worse when compromised in any way. I rarely have to point out the importance of planning to clients because it usually becomes so obvious that they reach the conclusion on their own.

The lesson is clear. If you want things to turn out well reliably, you have to set it up so that they can.

Those who heed the lesson go on to live much happier lives with food and in general. Those who don't, tend to remain stuck in an endless loop of self-deprivation alternating with self-abuse, seldom able to relax fully into their lives. It is entirely unnecessary to live this way. If you want something better, planning is the key.

Don't expect your emotional brain to embrace the notion of planning—it almost assuredly won't. Planning is not an emotional brain skill, and it involves a future beyond the emotional brain's perceptual range. Planning can only happen in the cortex, but needs to be done on the emotional brain's behalf and with top priority placed on the emotional brain's needs. As long as the emotional brain is kept adequately satisfied along the way (Chapter 23), the cortex is free to keep developing and carrying out the plans that will create a good future for the emotional brain to enjoy once it gets there.

Elements of Effective Planning

Good planning gets you the most enjoyment and best results that your personal circumstances allow, and in ways that align well with your natural tendencies. This means that you spend more time just living your life and less time fighting with yourself. Perhaps best of all, planning means that you reap all these rewards with the least possible effort.

Good planning should be simple, because complicated plans feel intimidating, are hard to execute correctly, and include too much room for error. Simple plans reduce the number and complexity of decisions that have to be made each day; they reduce stress while improving results.

The dilemma of whether to eat or not—and how much—is something we would rarely face out in the wild, so it's no wonder that we now find it exhausting and burdensome to have to consider such decisions all day long, every day. Planning is what enables us to scale the decision-making back to a level that is more manageable.

One example of a simple plan is to identify an easy, nutritious breakfast and just have that same breakfast every day. If you need a bit of variety, identify a few such breakfasts, make sure you always have the necessary ingredients on hand for at least two of them, and just have whichever one you prefer on a given day. Common mainstays are cereal (there are actually a few that are nutritious and tasty), eggs, oatmeal, fruit, yogurt, and smoothies, though leftovers from last night's nutritious dinner would work just as well if you're so inclined. The point is to find something which is easy and enjoyable, and which gives your body a strong start to the day. The end result is that you always get a good breakfast and never have to debate about the issue again if you don't want to.

Another simple plan is to decide on your meals for a week, figure out the shopping necessary to make those meals, and then make that your basic plan for each week. You'll be free to introduce more variety whenever you have the time and inclination to do so, but on the weeks when you don't have time, you can just default to the basic plan. It'll be easy to do, you'll know it well, and you'll stay well-fed with minimal decision-making and effort. Better yet, have some of your dinners planned to include extra for leftovers that can be used in lunches or frozen as individual servings for later use.

You don't need to spend endless hours in the kitchen each week to make this work. Part of your system is to determine—using that awesome cortex of yours—how to make it as easy as possible. This will take some experimentation and extra thought up front, but once you get it figured out, it becomes a simple matter of familiar follow-through.

Simple options like those described above have the advantage of allowing you to automate your food practices to some degree. Look for patterns that you like and which work well for you, then just keep repeating them. Do this enough to save time and emotional energy, but not so much that it feels boring and repetitive. Such patterns can become the core of your new system, giving you variety and creativity where it really matters to you, and a nutritious default option for when you don't feel like thinking about what to do.

Good planning makes it both easier to stay on track and harder to make damaging mistakes. Make it easy to eat nutritious food by assuring that you always have enough of it on hand in your home, restocking before you run out. It's always best to keep several options available so that if you do run out of something, you have a fallback plan or two. Or even three or four. Here's one example of what this can look like in actual practice.

Let's say the dinner you plan to cook for tonight is Plan A. If you don't feel like cooking or discover at the last minute that you're short a critical ingredient, Plan B might be the leftovers in the fridge from earlier this week, or some frozen leftovers from when you cooked at some time in the past. If none of that is available or appealing, Plan C could be some commercially prepared frozen entrees that you keep on hand for just this kind of situation, which you've carefully researched and have found to be nutritious enough to do in a pinch. Failing that, you have an easy Plan D if at some point, you researched canned options and brought home a few that have an acceptable nutritional profile and are tasty enough to be appealing.

If all those plans fail to meet your needs on a given day, maybe you'll consider a Plan E that involves a bowl of one of those nutritious boxed cereals that you keep around,[1] or perhaps you have some eggs on hand that can easily be whipped up as your Plan F.

You've just read an example of a primary plan with up to *five* backups that could be set up by anyone. All it takes to have a safety net that big is to plan for it, set it up, and then maintain it. Planning and initial setup take a bit of time, but once you have it in place, all you have to do is keep an eye on your various supplies to assure that you remain well-stocked.

The beauty of having a five- or six-layer system of redundancy is that—since life happens and you're going to end up out of some things now and then—you're assured of always still having a few workable options available. If you ever let *every* layer of your system go out of stock at the same time (other than in the context of an emergency), it shows that you need to be more mindful about monitoring your supplies.

It's important to maintain enough options so that in any given moment, you'll find one of them acceptable enough that you won't just call for takeout instead. You must have options that are *easy* and *enjoyable* so that your emotional brain will consider them at all, and *nutritious* enough to support the physical health you need for the life that you want.

Planning with several layers of fallback options is especially important for those who live in "food deserts," those urban and rural areas where fresh food is harder to get simply because the nearest grocery store is too far away to allow for frequent replenishment of home supplies. People in these areas are dependent on convenience stores for any spur-of-the-moment food needs, so their most accessible options are heavily oriented toward fat, sugar, salt, and other additives—the very foods that compromise health and detract from quality of life.[2]

Residents in these areas need to be the most careful planners of all since they don't have the luxury of just popping out to a fully stocked grocery store whenever they feel like it. While they can enjoy fresh foods in the days immediately after a major shopping trip, they need to rely heavily on items which can be stored for longer periods of time, whether in the freezer or on the shelf.

Nutritious, shelf-stable options include whole-grain cereals, dried beans and lentils, brown rice, and grains like bulgur, barley, quinoa, and millet for use in home recipes. With a bit of comparison shopping, you can find some canned goods that have a minimum of additives and which are a valuable addition to any home pantry.[3]

The home freezer is an especially important part of the plan for residents in food deserts, making it possible not only to stock up on a variety of frozen meats and produce, but also to make and freeze individual portions of home-cooked recipes for easy future use.

By the way, if you have the good fortune to live where fresh food is readily available but would simply prefer not to shop very often, you might like using the strategies that work for those who live in food deserts. Whether you do it by necessity or choice, you'll be able to keep a steady supply of nutritious food in your home while minimizing the time you spend in the grocery store.

Doing Your Homework

Good planning means doing some research up front when necessary so that later follow-through will be simple and straight-forward. When stocking your home as described above, you'll need to do some label-reading at first in order to determine which canned and packaged items meet your requirements for becoming part of your standard inventory. Once you've identified those items, they become familiar entries on your shopping list and you just grab them at the store without having to think about the choice any more.

If a product you use gets reformulated in any way, you'll need to analyze it again just as you did in the beginning because it may have been changed in ways that no longer meet your requirements. You'll also have to do an evaluation of your alternate choices any time one of your stand-by foods has to go out of rotation, whether it's because you no longer wish to use it, your grocery store has stopped stocking it, or the manufacturer has taken it out of production. Other than those exceptions, once you've gotten through the initial round of reading and comparing labels, you won't need to do much of it going forward.

When it comes to eating out, your homework involves researching restaurants and menu options online before you go. Restaurants are highly triggering places where we all need to spend less time, frankly. When we do go, we need to be prepared.

It is far easier to peruse a menu at your leisure, without distractions, than it is to do so there in the restaurant with its triggering sights, sounds, and smells. You can take your time selecting the entrees you find most appealing, then see how they stack up in terms of calories, fat content, and sodium loading.

It is important to do this research because the numbers can be truly shocking. When you find an innocent-sounding item to have over 1000 mg of sodium, for example, it's a lot easier to move on to a different selection. Eventually, you'll either find something that offers a balance of enjoyment and nutrition that you find acceptable, or you'll realize that particular restaurant is just best avoided altogether.

Another example of doing your homework is to find out ahead of time what will be served when you will be a guest in someone's home or at a social event. This will give you time to get used to the idea of what you'll see when you get there, and also to develop some strategies to help you have the best experience when the time comes.

Remembering the Time Element

Many of us now lead lives that feel rushed, with multiple demands on our time and many obligations to meet. We have jobs, kids with dense activity schedules, homes that require ongoing upkeep, friendships to maintain, and various appointments to keep. I've seen many personal calendars that are just blackened with ink, showing multiple commitments for most days of the week.

It is easy in the midst of all this busyness to forget to leave time for grocery shopping, food preparation, occasional nutrition research, and regular physical activity. You need all of these activities and you need them with some consistency if you hope to get and stay in control with food. If you don't plan time for them, they will happen haphazardly or not at all, and you'll never escape the chaos.

Planning is something that any of us can do more effectively. Doing it poorly will get you better results than not doing it at all, so the learning curve is risk-free. You'll get better and more efficient at it with practice, which means it will gradually take less time and effort. It will always take *some* time and effort, but it can become so automatic that you hardly notice you're doing it. While the effort will be something that you notice less and less, the benefits will keep you at your strongest and happiest every single day.

Chapter 28
Risk Management: The Zones

We can't change the fact that modern life is inherently hazardous to the emotional brain, but we can do a lot to mitigate the level of challenge that we each personally face. When you are more aware of what increases your risk, you are in a position to reduce it when possible and manage it more effectively when necessary. It helps to have a way to identify the various levels of risk, making it easier to recognize them as they occur and to respond accordingly. What follows is one such system of identification.

1. Red Zone—You've lost control; regrettable behavior is a given.

2. Orange Zone—You haven't lost control yet, but you're just hanging on by a thread.

3. Yellow Zone—You are comfortably in control as long as you remain mindful and choose with care.

4. Green Zone—You are effortlessly in control.

You're in the red zone when your emotional brain is triggered intensely enough to have locked out the cortex. You feel overpowering urges, and controlled decision-making is no longer possible. You're going to behave in a way that you'll later regret and you know it, but you're powerless to stop it. Because loss of free will is an essential characteristic of the red zone, it must be avoided whenever possible.

You can be triggered into the red zone in many different ways that are specific to you as an individual. Typical examples include restaurant buffets, birthday parties, holiday meals, food gifts, treats showing up at work, having triggering food at home, or simply allowing yourself to get so hungry that you'll grab the first and easiest option you can find. You're more vulnerable to slipping into the red zone when you're tired, distracted, upset, or haven't planned well enough to have easy, nutritious choices readily available. There are probably certain foods that launch you instantly into the red zone as soon as you see them.

Nobody fares well in the red zone because, by definition, we've already lost control if we're there. The only choice is to avoid it. On the bright side, most red zone exposure is self-inflicted due to poor setup, which means that most of it can be avoided with planning. If your life is set up in ways that result in a lot of red, you need to make some changes because success is impossible if you don't.

The reality of our world is such that even with the most conscientious setup, you're still going to trip into some red now and then. All that's left at that point is to do your best, try to minimize the damage, and get to safer ground as quickly as you can. This will be easier if you've considered some emergency strategies ahead of time, because the nature of red is that you won't have any problem-solving ability once you're in the midst of it.

You're in the orange zone when you are able to maintain your emotional balance around food only with great, focused effort. You have to concentrate so much on maintaining control that it interferes significantly with your ability to enjoy what is otherwise going on around you. You haven't lost control yet, but you're one wrong move away from doing so. This is exhausting to keep up for long and since exhaustion is one of the risks that can tip you into red, you need to spend as little time as possible in orange.

Like red, most orange is self-inflicted but some is unavoidable. The key is to eliminate it where you can, and then to limit as much as possible your time in that which remains. Most red is preceded by orange, so orange is your last chance to have at least a bit of cortex available to make the best of things. Again, you won't have much problem-solving ability in this state because you'll be so occupied with just trying to maintain control. If you've figured out some strategies ahead of time though, you may be able to remember that they exist and to use them while you can still think at least a little bit.

The yellow zone is a considerably happier state of affairs. Keeping your balance with food still requires some attention and effort, but the amount required is very manageable since your emotional brain is not being heavily triggered. This leaves you free to enjoy whatever else you're doing while keeping one corner of your awareness trained on your choices with food. In those moments when your emotional brain starts to spin up a bit, you are able to redirect yourself without much trouble since you're doing it before the emotional brain develops much momentum. You can spend many hours in yellow if you have to because it's not very tiring, but it's nice afterward when you can get yourself into a setting in which it is safe to fully relax.

The green zone is where we would spend all of our time if only we could, because it means the emotional brain is fully settled and content, feeling no impulsivity. In such a state, you are free to simply relax and enjoy your surroundings, not having to focus on mindful awareness if you don't want to.

Green—as it relates to eating—is a given if you're in a setting where food is not an option, since nothing solves the issue of self-control quite as effectively as simple lack of opportunity. You can get green zone time in lots of other ways, however.

For example, you're likely to be in the green whenever you engage in any activity that is simply incompatible with eating, like washing dishes, needlework, sorting laundry, yardwork, playing with your kids outside, cleaning, tending flowers, or doing anything else that requires keeping your hands free of food. You can also enjoy green zone time by engaging in activities or challenges that are so mentally stimulating or engrossing that food simply doesn't occur to you while you're busy.

There is a way to enjoy green zone time even in the presence of food opportunity; it happens whenever you are around *only* those foods and circumstances that you know you can easily manage. In such settings, you get to simply enjoy the moment, including the food, and to feel good about how you're handling yourself. Best of all, you get to feel very pleased afterward with the choices you ultimately made.

The green zone is where you will find emotional peace and freedom from having to work at self-control. The more you plan your life to turn out this way, the more enjoyable it becomes.

As mentioned in the last chapter, we each have a finite amount of willpower available each day for focus and control with food. It is enough to get us through any day that is primarily yellow and green, because yellow requires only a manageable amount of willpower and green actually replenishes it. Orange and red, on the other hand, drain it very quickly, which is why those situations need to be avoided as much as possible.

Hours or days spent in orange or red are damaging in any event, but the greater hazard is that such times tend to become a vicious cycle. The more regularly you have high-risk days with bad outcomes, the lower your available focus for each new day—the harder it is, the harder it gets. Fortunately, the negative spiral can be broken at any time with better planning and setup. The sooner you do it, the easier it will be.

Alternatively, the more green time you get, the greater your available focus for each new day because green actually creates energy and strength. The better it is, the better it gets. This is a relaxing and rewarding way to live that will only happen through planning; the work of planning is not difficult or terribly time-consuming, but does need to be generally consistent.

Factors That Affect Your Risk

We all face food challenges each day. The degree to which we struggle with those challenges depends on the zone we're in, and that depends mostly on how we prepare ourselves ahead of time, as you'll see in the scenarios that follow on the next few pages.

In each one, where you end up on the spectrum of risk depends on how you manage the variables that are in your control. The lines of demarcation between zones in these examples are generic and probably fairly accurate for many people, but your personal experience may vary. Regardless of where the boundaries between zones fall for you, the fact is that in most situations, you have the power to make control with food either easier or harder for yourself, at least to some degree.

Scenario #1: A Trigger Food is Calling Your Name

RED	The food is ready to eat and nearby, where you can see it.
ORANGE	The food is ready to eat and nearby, out of sight.
YELLOW	None of the food is on hand, but you keep thinking about it and have no good way to distract yourself.
GREEN	None of the food is on hand, and you have other ways to keep yourself occupied.

When you have an urge for a particular food, the variables you deal with are the physical proximity of the food and the availability of other activities. The closer you are to the food, the more likely your emotional brain is to be triggered into impulsive action. Greater physical distance works in your favor.

It also helps to know of some other ways to redirect yourself when food urges come. Lacking other things to do, you might just go out to get the food even though your home is safely free of it. The key to maximizing green in this instance is to have your home free of foods you can't resist, and to always have some other ways to occupy yourself that are acceptable to your emotional brain.

Scenario #2: You're in the Grocery Store

RED	You have no list and are prone to impulse buying.
ORANGE	You're with someone who is impulsive.
ORANGE	You're tired, frustrated, hungry, or rushed.
YELLOW	You're with someone whose presence helps you to maintain control.
YELLOW	You're feeling centered, rested, and strong.
GREEN	You have a list that you reliably stick to, and it includes no trigger foods.

Going to the grocery store involves more variables than you might realize. Are you going in with a game plan or not? Or you going with someone (like a child or a fellow overeater) who encourages impulsivity or with someone who helps you to stay focused? Are you in a calm, balanced frame of mind, or are you rushed and distracted?

These are all variables that you usually have time to tilt more in your favor if you plan ahead. If you don't, you'll be left with no choice but to deal with the task the best you can when the time comes. This means that more than likely, it will be your emotional brain doing the shopping.

Scenario #3: Someone is Pressuring You to Take a Trigger Food Home

RED	The person is a loved one and you're not very assertive.
ORANGE	The person is a loved one with whom you can be assertive.
ORANGE	The person is an acquaintance and you're not very assertive.
YELLOW	The person is an acquaintance with whom you can be assertive.
RED	You've taken the food home.

The scenario above refers to those times when the food you're being pressured to accept is food that is likely to threaten your self-control at home, and which you'd rather not take. The element that you can't control is the closeness of your relationship with the person who is trying to give you the food. It's important to understand that the closer the relationship is, the more you will feel obligated to accept the food no matter how much you don't want it.

This isn't hopeless, however, because there is a variable that you *can* influence, and that's your ability to be assertive. When you know you're likely to be faced with this challenge, you can mentally rehearse ahead of time how you wish to respond.

For the times when it comes up unexpectedly, it can help to establish an automatic default of declining, rather than trying to think on your feet while under pressure. If you do decline, be prepared to repeat the polite refusal several times over, because people who pressure others to take food don't readily take no for an answer.

If you think that saying no will create too much relational discord, another variable in your control is what you do with the food after accepting it. I've known many people who have thrown it out on the way home, and none who have regretted doing so. Your emotional brain will start rumbling when the food is initially presented, but will be doing so much more intensely if you take it home. The easiest strategy is just to keep the food from ever getting there.

Scenario #4: Coworkers Suggest Fast Food for Lunch

RED	You didn't bring any lunch of your own.
ORANGE	You brought a lunch, but you weren't looking forward to it anyway.
YELLOW	You eat your own enjoyable lunch alongside your coworkers.
GREEN	You eat your own enjoyable lunch somewhere else, away from the sights and smells of the group meal.

When a coworker says something like, "Hey, how about if we all go in on pizza?" the variables involve how much you planned ahead, but also how you feel about time with your coworkers and what your practical options are for where you can spend your lunchtime.

The scenario is not meant to imply that you must be a hermit and miss out on valued time with friends in favor of having greater control with food. In fact, it shows a realistic case of multiple priorities. Your happiness and quality of life are dramatically affected by how balanced you stay with food, but also by time spent with supportive friends. The challenge is how to get the best of both worlds.

It's important to notice the things you can do to make the food part less stressful if you wish, and to understand that when you choose to eat with friends who are indulging in food you're trying to avoid, you'll have to work a bit harder at keeping your eating under control. It's about balancing your needs in the way that keeps you the happiest and strongest overall.

Scenario #5: Someone Brought
Goodies to Share at Work

RED	The goodies are close enough to your work area that you can see and smell them all day.
ORANGE	They're not in your work area, but you have to walk by them regularly.
YELLOW	You know where the goodies are, but they're not near enough for you to see or smell them. You're able to avoid that area until they're gone.
GREEN	You're able to work in a different location until the goodies are gone.

When goodies are sitting out at work, you're dealing with proximity issues, sensory triggering, the human tendency to mirror the behavior of others who are eating, and possible social pressure to conform.

These potent forces are all aligned against the one variable you *might* have any control over, which is the physical distance you maintain from the food. Of all the places we experience food pressure now more than ever before, the workplace may be the most damaging. We spend a great deal of our time there and if food shows up in our space, we are not free to leave.

It's important to do whatever you can to create some distance, trying to create a safe buffer for your emotional brain in any way possible. This may include being more assertive about treat foods not being kept in your immediate vicinity, and perhaps even questioning the workplace practices that subject everyone to so much food pressure.

Challenging those practices is important for the same reason we once challenged—and changed—the presence of second-hand smoke in the workplace: health and lives are at stake. In the meantime, many workplaces—in the name of good times, shared fun, and not wasting food—will continue to undermine the health of their employees by making it impossible to escape the situations that trigger so many of us to lose control of our eating.

Scenario #6: You're Tired from Your Long Day and It's Time for Dinner

RED	You didn't plan dinner and there's not much in the house that you'd enjoy.
ORANGE	You didn't plan dinner but there are options on hand that would take some time and trouble.
YELLOW	You didn't plan dinner, but have some quality options on hand that you like and which can be prepared easily on the spur of the moment.
GREEN	You had an enjoyable dinner set up for easy preparation, so now it's just a matter of following through.

The variables you're confronted with at the end of a tiring day are how much time and effort it will take to acquire a dinner that you like.

Being tired, you won't have much determination or patience; it will take very little to tip the emotional brain into taking control. If you haven't set up some easy, tasty, nutritious options at home, you're more likely to go for the easy, tasty, not-so-nutritious options available via takeout, delivery, or eating out.

Scenario #7: You're Eating Out

RED	You're with others who overeat when out.
RED	You've "saved room" so you can enjoy dinner more.
RED	You're at an unfamiliar restaurant with many triggering options.
RED	You're going to make your selection based on "what looks good" once you get there. You have no plan.
ORANGE	You're at a restaurant with some quality options, but also some very triggering ones. You have no plan.
YELLOW	You researched the menu ahead of time and made your decision before arriving. You don't even need to look at the menu when you get there.
GREEN	You know the restaurant well and reliably make choices there that are enjoyable without triggering you into loss of control.

Oh, where to start? For anyone with overeating issues, eating out is a high-risk activity under the best of circumstances. Restaurants are highly triggering places, purposely designed to get you to eat as much as possible. Then there's the question of whether or not your dinner companions tend to overeat. If they do, you will likely do the same as you all mirror each other's behavior. If you've made a point of arriving extra-hungry, you're more likely to choose impulsively once you arrive.

Then there's the question of the restaurant you're going to on this occasion. Have you done your homework prior to arriving? Is it a place where you know you can find some options that will be enjoyable and give you no cause for regret afterward? Have you positioned yourself to be able to *make* those choices once you get there?

As noted in Chapter 3, we eat out more than ever before. This means we frequently and voluntarily subject ourselves to triggering food environments in which the risk of losing control is very high. The obvious first line of defense is to spend less time in such environments; the second line of defense is to reduce the risks as much as possible through careful research and planning.

Your Primary Zones and Your Odds of Success

If you spend a lot of your time in the orange and red zones—as is the case with most of my clients when they begin therapy—food will remain a love/hate torment in your life. I have yet to meet an individual who can maintain self-control under such circumstances.

If you live mostly in the yellow and orange zones, things are marginally better. You can white-knuckle your way to some success, but much of your energy must remain focused on preventing loss of control rather than on enjoying your life.

Life quality spikes dramatically once you start spending your time primarily in the yellow and green zones. Self-control is easier and therefore more reliable, which means you get to relax more. You get to spend a large portion of your available energy on your actual life, rather than on food and whether or not you're doing okay with it.

While a life lived fully in the green zone would be ideal, it's not possible unless you spend your time only in your own properly stocked home and in spaces managed exclusively by others who share your goals and values about food. Since that is unlikely, the reasonable goal is to get your life as far into the yellow/green zone as possible, expecting to have some wobbly spots of orange and red every now and then.

If you manage this, you can expect to still struggle a bit on occasion, but only in certain, limited circumstances. Most of the time, your life with food will simply be peaceful and satisfying. It's a nice way to live, and the only reliable way to keep your balance with food for a lifetime.

Any choice that brings more yellow and green time into your life is likely to be a positive one. If you're not sure where to start, consider some of the basics like reducing your exposure to triggering situations, spending more time in activities and in places where eating is not an easy option, cooking at home more, leading a more active lifestyle, planning for the better outcomes you desire, developing non-food ways to meet more of your needs, and focusing your time with friends and family more on shared activities and less on food.

The Dilemma of the Great Cook

It was noted in Chapter 3 that many people now lack basic cooking skills, but there is an important exception to this, since some of us are actually great cooks. Others of us are at least capable of preparing meals that—if not nutritionally optimal—are really delicious and fun to eat. If you're capable of making wonderful food, you must take care not to use your skills in ways that create more orange and red time in your world or that of your loved ones. Just because you *can* create irresistible food doesn't mean it's a good idea. If you want food to be a source of enjoyment for your family without the unwanted baggage of regrettable overeating, you may need to dial it back a bit.

Good food is a positive and relaxing experience. You eat it, enjoy it, and then stop eating with relative ease and calm once you've had a reasonable amount. Food that is *irresistible*—most often due to extra sweeteners, sodium, fats, or other additives—is a complicated experience with an element of torment. You eat it, love it in a crazed way, fight with yourself to eat less than you want, and ultimately overeat enough to feel regret afterwards.

There's a similar issue with portion size. The natural tendency is to eat whatever is in front of you, so it's simple and easy when all that's in front of you is an amount that will be enjoyable without causing harm. You just enjoy the food until it's gone and then shift your attention elsewhere when you're done. Oversized portions, on the other hand, force you into the frantic internal debate about how much to have and when to stop, followed most often by a feeling of having gone too far. It's a surprisingly stressful experience, all in all.

If you want your home to be a safe place for the emotional brains of all who live there, it's important to present food that allows those brains to remain comfortably in control. The secret to that is keeping both palatability and portion size within limits that everyone can easily handle, recognizing that there is interplay between the two. The more triggering the food, the more important it is to be careful about portion size.

The solution is to cook in smaller quantities overall, portioning the food to keep the calorie load of each serving at a healthful level. Smaller portions make it easier to stop eating at the right time anyway, especially if there's not a lot of food left for seconds. This may not be the way you're accustomed to cooking, but it's a way to help yourself and your loved ones to maintain easier self-control while enjoying your fabulous food.

Managing Your Zones

Zones are a function of more than just the situation you're in and how much you did or did not plan ahead. The zone you experience is also a result of your internal state, such as what mood you're in, how tired or distracted you are, and even how you feel physically. Because this varies from day to day, it's a good idea to get in the habit of noticing what zone you're in at any given time, and remaining on the lookout for ways to shift yourself to a safer zone whenever possible.

Ideally, using the magic of planning and strategic setup, you'd find a clever way to convert every potentially red or orange situation into something easier and more enjoyable. That will be possible much of the time, but realistically, there will be some situations you just can't make safe enough. Given the overwhelmingly food-centric nature of our society—and therefore most of your family, friends, and neighbors— there will always be some events you want to attend even though you know full well that the food will be a major struggle for you.

When you knowingly go into a red or orange situation, the best fallback strategy is to go in with a clear plan for how to keep yourself as safe as possible. This plan starts with when you'll arrive and how long you'll stay. If you're a sucker for appetizers and you know they'll be present in abundance, for example, you might plan on arriving closer to dinnertime so that you won't be exposed to them for very long. If you know in your heart that the longer you're there, the more you'll eat, you might set up some outside plan that forces you to leave by a certain time.

You can arrive with a clear set of social goals for your time, to give you something other than the food to think about. Perhaps there are certain people you want to be sure to talk to and certain conversations you want to make sure you have. If there will be people present whom you don't know very well, you could make a point of learning more about them. Such goals will strengthen your relationships and social connections (always a good thing) in addition to nudging food off the center stage of your attention.

Some of my clients have benefitted from making a list of such goals and taking it with them to the event, whether on their smartphone or simply on a scrap of paper in their pocket. If they feel themselves starting to focus too much on the food, they remember the list and choose an idea from it so they can redirect their attention and reduce the pressure they're feeling about the food. It's remarkable how well this works.

Your plan might also include where you will be throughout the event, with an emphasis on keeping as much physical and visual distance as possible between you and the food. Alternatively, if you are at an event in someone's home, you might benefit from keeping yourself busy assisting the hosts so that you aren't just hanging around munching. The hosts will appreciate it a great deal, and you'll be happier with having maintained your balance a bit better.

In any situation with potential exposure to red or orange levels of challenge, try to be aware of your most vulnerable points and be especially strategic about those. Avoid triggers as much as you can and minimize your time around those that you can't avoid altogether, keeping yourself otherwise occupied as much as possible. As always, look for ways to create or move to easier and safer circumstances as soon as you can.

Chapter 29
Being Part of the Solution: Support of Others

This book is dedicated to the understanding and management of overeating, but we can't fully address this for ourselves if we continue to remain part of the problem for others.

The social overemphasis on food that was described in Chapter 2 is not just a matter of the people around us. *We* are part of that environment for others as well; our actions have great bearing on the degree to which others struggle with orange and red zones of risk.

Looking Out for Our Loved Ones

We live in a high-pressure food environment because the vast majority of us actively and continuously contribute to it. We do it to conform to social norms and expectations, and we do it because we want to be generous to others. We also do it because the food industry spends billions of dollars annually on marketing campaigns that keep food ever-present in our minds.

It is essential to remember that these forces act upon us at all times. If we remain conscious of this, we can each begin to choose differently, gradually reshaping our culture in ways that benefit us all.

This kind of change has to start at home, and that brings us right back to the emotional brain. Once again, there is an important lesson to be found in how we relate to our pets. As previously discussed, our pets lack the brain development to understand the hazards of today's world and as a result, their safety depends on us using our cortex on their behalf. Fortunately for them, this is something we do quite well … except when it comes to feeding time.

Pets are often overfed, sometimes literally to death, by people who are otherwise diligent and dedicated caretakers. This is due in large part to the fact that feeding our pets is very rewarding—for us. It obviously makes them happy, and we like seeing them happy because we love them. They do silly and entertaining things when they get excited about food, which can be a lot of fun. In fact, it's like a little party every time it happens, which is very rewarding to our emotional brain.

And that's where things can start to go wrong. You might enjoy the process so much—*Look how cute he is, dancing around for his food!*—that feeding time becomes more about your own enjoyment than about the health and welfare of your pet.

Your cortex would dole out food based solely on maximizing your pet's health, while your emotional brain doles it out based on having a great party. Leave your emotional brain in charge of feeding your pet for long enough, and your pet will end up at risk for many of the same diseases your doctor might be warning *you* about.

Your emotional brain is wholly unqualified for the job of managing food for *anyone* in an environment of abundance. Only your cortex can sort out the various opportunities and risks to come up with an approach to food that maximizes both enjoyment and health. If you make food decisions for yourself *or for anyone else* from your emotional brain, it will result in decisions that maximize immediate reward (whether yours or theirs) at the expense of long-term health.

This has serious ramifications for how we feed our families, because we love seeing *them* have a good time, too. In fact, most of my clients eventually express concern that if they make changes at home in support of more controlled and nutritious eating for themselves, it will take something of value away from their families: *Why should they have to suffer just because I have food problems? That's not fair to them.*

This reveals an enormous blind spot, given that we're talking about the products that cause *most* people to lose control of their behavior, sooner or later. When you lose control of your behavior, you lose the ability to act in your own best interests. You also lose the power to protect yourself from harm. This is terribly risky in any context.

If you're reading this book, it has probably already happened to you with certain foods and beverages. If you continue to keep those products in your home, they are likely to have the same effect on most or all of your family members, if they haven't already.

Even if others in the family don't feel the addictive pull as you have, the fact remains that these products—unless used in careful moderation—have a very negative impact on health. Nearly 40% of the calories consumed by kids in the US today are devoid of nutritional benefit while including disproportional amounts of solid fats and added sugars (pizza and soda figure heavily in this).[1] This is not working, given that our children are increasingly subject to serious medical problems caused by poor nutrition and obesity.

The best thing you can do for your family is to lead the way, showing by example what it looks like and how it works to take good care of yourself, nutritionally and otherwise. You can be the one who shows them how to get creative about non-food ways to show love, have fun, pass the time, deal with stress, and all the rest.

This will be challenging, given that they are growing up in a world where overeating of non-food products is the norm. That makes it all the more important for you to do what you can to maintain a home environment where it is easy to stay healthy.

You and your needs are not an inconvenience to your family. You and the changes you need to make are the best chance your family has at figuring out how to navigate an environment so fraught with peril when it comes to food.

The Dilemma of Excess and Unwanted Food

If you decide to purge your home of food products that undermine the wellbeing of your family, you'll be faced with the question of what to do with all of it. This won't be the only time you'll have to think about this.

Depending on the time of year, you'll occasionally find yourself in possession of pounds of unused Halloween candy, a surplus of baked holiday goodies, or even just leftovers from your last big party. All you'll know is that having the stuff sitting around your home is a setup for trouble, and that you need it to be somewhere else as soon as possible.

Now you'll be faced with two imperatives: the need to get rid of the food and the need to keep it from going to waste. Giving it away would seem to be the perfect solution, and that's what most people do. Sometimes they give it to relatives, friends, or neighbors, but the single most popular destination for unwanted food is the workplace. Regardless of where the food ends up, the important thing is that it's gone. Problem solved. But wait ...

If most of the people around you struggle with overeating (Chapter 1), then you've probably reduced your own risk by shifting it onto someone else who can't handle it any better than you can. Most people do this. This is part of what makes our world as food-pressured as it is, and this is what we need to change.

Shifting unwanted food into the workplace is an especially damaging practice because, as noted in the last chapter, people in the workplace are a captive audience. I hear stories every week of people who—due to the location of their work area relative to where the food shows up—are forced to see it, smell it, and witness others eating it all day.

Combine this with the pressure and frustrations of an average work day, and you've just created an orange-to-red level situation for a group of people who have no choice but to stay in place and struggle with it for hours on end. Most will eventually succumb to the food you've put in their space and—having now blown it all day at work—will go on to keep bingeing at home because their day feels like a total loss anyway.

If we want a less food-pressured world where we don't have to be so watchful and careful all the time, then we each need to do our own part in creating it. That begins with neutralizing risk rather than shifting it onto others.

The best way to neutralize risk is to avoid it in the first place. Buy less food. Prepare less food. Eat out less frequently. Bring less food into your life to start with so that the problem of excess is prevented before it develops.

Because so much of our economy and culture centers on the production and distribution of food, however, you'll almost certainly find yourself dealing with excess sometimes despite your most determined efforts. Unless you know someone who will truly benefit from the food when those times come, the only reasonable alternative is to dispose of it.

Most people balk at this because it feels wrong, but when you're dealing with too much food, there's no good option. It may seem wasteful to discard it, but it's *harmful* to foist it onto someone else who has no more use for it than you do.

Disposing of excess food is simply the lesser of evils. If you hate the idea of doing that, the only solution is to keep it from entering your world in the first place.

Chapter 30
Living More, Eating Less

Much of the difficulty we have with food today stems from the fact that we have made it too important in our lives. When you have an abundance of something—anything—it is natural to make use of it in as many ways as possible. We have an abundance of food, and it seems to apply handily to a wide variety of uses.

If you want something to do, eating feels like an activity. If you want to enjoy yourself, food provides several forms of sensory pleasure. If you don't like how you feel, eating is a pleasant distraction. If you can't concentrate, you can focus your attention on food. If you want to share time with someone, sharing food is a safe choice because no matter how else we differ as individuals, we all eat. If you want to celebrate something special, food is the star attraction of virtually every social tradition we have for such times. If you want to extend a kindness or simply let someone know you care about them, a gift of food is an easy and universally recognized way in which to do it.

Food has become our most versatile multi-use tool, gradually taking the place of many other things we used to do and think about before it became so readily available. It would be nice if using food the way we now do actually *worked*, but it doesn't. This way of life is making too many of us sick. It's making too many of us clinically depressed and dooming too many of us to years of needless physical limitation and suffering. It is causing too many premature deaths.

We can avoid much of this grief by returning food to a more proportional place in our lives. This means continuing to enjoy it, share it, and look forward to it, but doing so *within our physical limits*. When we start making other things more important in our lives again, there will naturally be less emphasis on food. This will help all of us with self-control, in addition to giving us a richer variety of ways in which to enjoy ourselves and take care of our emotional needs.

You might think that after being dependent on food to meet so many needs for so long, it would be hard for most people to imagine what to do instead. The first time I invited seminar participants to come up with some non-food ways to meet common social and emotional needs, I did so with some trepidation because I wasn't sure how well they would do.

As it turned out, I needn't have worried. I've found that when people take the time really to *think* about alternatives, especially when several people are able to brainstorm together, they always come up with plenty of ideas. It is an inspiring and heartwarming process to witness as everyone starts feeling creative, energetic, and excited in ways that they have not experienced when focusing on food-centered plans and ideas.

I've since heard from many who have gone on to use those fresh ideas in their own lives, and all have felt greatly enriched for having done so. In fact, they've all emphasized how much more they *enjoyed* themselves in general. These comments are typical: "The kids loved it ... We had a great time ... It felt really good to do this ... It was the best family get-together we've had in a long time." They tell me these stories with big, relaxed smiles. They look happy.

This reveals perhaps the most important consequence of overemphasizing food in our lives. We now use eating in place of other personal and relational practices that would be far more nourishing to the spirit, and the spirits of many have been left impoverished as a result. I speak every day with people who have been trying for years to fill that void with food, becoming emptier inside as their bodies become sicker, bigger, and more unwieldy.

This is another compelling reason to give food a smaller role in our lives. It's not just about reducing caloric intake, although that is a result we happen to need desperately. The more important outcome is that the attention you turn away from food will be turned *toward* thoughts and activities that are far better at enriching your life and feeding your spirit. It's an amazing win-win.

It will be easier to begin directing more of your time and attention in other ways if you first clarify the main reasons that you've been overusing food. You are likely to find that most of it boils down to pursuing reward, seeking comfort, or simply looking for a way to be occupied, often for the purpose of escaping inner emotional noise.

I have asked numerous clients and seminar participants for their ideas on non-food ways to satisfy these needs. I have been aggregating their responses for some time now, organizing the ideas based on the needs they most readily address. As you consider the options below and perhaps come up with more of your own, remember that this isn't simply about eating less. It's about replacing food in the areas of your life where other alternatives will work better for you anyway. You'll probably be amazed when you discover (or remember) the sheer bliss of some of the simplest things. Have fun exploring.

Rewards and Treats

- Read something for pleasure
- Have a soothing cup of tea
- Put on music you love and really listen to it
- Take a bath or shower just to relax
- Watch one of your favorite movies or try out a new one
- Light some candles
- Do your nails
- Sit outside on a pleasant day

- Arrange a kid-free shopping trip
- Get a new book
- Try some new music
- Get your hair cut and styled
- Get a haircut with a hot lather neck shave
- Get a facial
- Get that new tool you've been eyeing up for your workbench
- Get a massage
- Special outings (zoo, museum, etc.)

Comfort and Relief

- Prayer
- Meditation
- Yoga
- Stretch for a few minutes
- Sit out at night and watch the stars
- Hug someone
- Work on a puzzle

- Knit or crochet
- Counted cross-stitch
- Paint by numbers
- Paint or sketch freehand
- Crossword puzzle
- Doodle (have a look at www.zentangle.com for something different)

Comfort and Relief (continued)

- Use a coloring book for grown-ups
- Play a musical instrument
- Cuddle, groom, or play with a pet
- Look at treasured photos
- Call, message, or get together with a friend
- Read poetry
- Read inspirational material
- Listen to inspirational material
- Write in your personal journal
- Write a list of reasons to be grateful
- Take a walk on a wooded trail
- Go fishing, or just sit at the shore and watch the water
- Do "your thing"—your favorite hobby

Other Ways to Pass Some Time

- Do some minor decluttering where you'll enjoy the results the most.
- Exercise in a way that fits or lifts your mood.
- Watch funny videos.
- Make a plan with a friend or loved one that you can look forward to.
- Consider a personal goal that you could meet in a couple of months. List the steps you can start taking now to reach it.
- Get a small surprise gift for someone.
- Attend a class for something you've wanted to try.
- Volunteer for a cause that energizes you.
- Play a game with someone.
- Go out to a movie, concert, play, or other live event.
- Take a scenic ride on country roads.
- Make a point of visiting someone who is probably lonely.
- Explore a museum or other local attraction.

Other Ways to Pass Some Time (continued)

- Go for a relaxing walk-and-talk with a friend, or one of your kids.

- Perform random or anonymous acts of kindness.

- Give a handwritten note of appreciation to someone who won't be expecting it.

- Take a walk somewhere new.

- Read outside, at home or at a nearby lake or park.

- Go for a walk at a local park or walking trail.

- Do your usual walking route in the opposite direction, noticing what's different from this new perspective.

- Go for a bicycle ride.

- Go to a playground and swing.

- Fly a kite.

- Play outside with your kids.

- Try some hiking trails.

- Go fishing or paddling.

- Take your dog for a walk.

- Projects like sewing, needlework, woodworking, leatherwork.

- Putter in your yard or garden.

- Putter in your garage or at your workbench.

- Detail your car.

There is another way in which many of us overuse food, and that is in gifting to others, whether we do it as part of a special occasion or as a simple, spontaneous gesture of affection. We do this for a variety of reasons, chief among them being that gifts of food are easy and can be inexpensive. Because everyone eats, food seems to work as a gift for almost anyone: the person you don't know well but wish to acknowledge in some way; the person with whom you share only a casual or business relationship; the person who has everything.

Food is often used as an easy-out kind of gift, but that's not always the case. It can be a deeply personal gift, made with your own hands in your own kitchen, given with warmth and love to people you cherish deeply. There's something to be said for this in our increasingly impersonal world. It is a lovely ritual originating in times and circumstances radically different from our realities of today.

Regardless of the motivation behind gifts of food, they are now given in a context which is different and more complicated than anything we've experienced before. Few people need or even *want* more of the treat food that is most often given this way, as evidenced by how often such food gets passed off on others in an effort to get rid of it.

Many of us struggle with self-control when faced with such gifts, and struggling is an unwanted, unpleasant experience. Many of us now have health problems as a direct result of having eaten too much of that kind of food already, yet continue to be pelted with gifts that will assuredly increase our medical risk, sometimes with nonsensical directives like, "Well, just don't eat it all at once." We commonly reason that it's healthy to "live a little" for special occasions, but it's not "a little." We're already doing it quite regularly.

Nobody feels like they're living well when they can't walk anywhere without gasping for breath, are told that some toes need to be amputated, or have a heart attack or stroke. Suffering does come at some point if you ignore these realities for long enough, and I have to yet to speak with anyone who says it was worth it.

This is not to say we must banish all treat foods from our lives, which is good since few of us would consider giving them up altogether anyway. Most of us will work instead at figuring out how to keep some of them in the picture enough for enjoyment, but not enough to compromise physical health. That's a tricky balance to find, and it's a highly individual calculation which changes over time with age. It's one that each of us can make much more easily if we are making all of our *own* choices without the outside interference of unsolicited gifts of food.

Gifting with food can be done without risk of negative impact only if it is done with communication and forethought. This means assuring well ahead of time that the recipient actually wants the food *and* has no concerns about it. Assume nothing.

It would be overkill to have that kind of conversation when it comes to small gifts and relationships that aren't very personal, so the easiest solution is simply to default to giving something other than food. If you do, you'll be helping to reduce the food pressure with which we all live, and that will be a good thing. The ideas below represent the combined wisdom of numerous therapy group members and seminar participants; they should give you a good start.

Non-Food Gifts

- Reusable shopping bag
- Candles
- Book
- Assortment of teas
- CD
- DVD
- Scarf
- Flowers or a plant
- Book marks
- Small flashlight for key chain
- Crafts
- Pet-related items
- Picture frame
- Calendar
- Note pads
- Lottery tickets
- Magazine subscription
- Bath oil/shower gel/soap/lotion/etc.
- Cutting from one of your own plants, in a special gift pot
- Card with a note of appreciation or affection
- Books, toys, stickers, etc. for kids

Gifts of Time

- Babysitting
- Social plans with someone who is lonely
- Yardwork
- Snow removal
- Read to someone with poor vision
- Wash/wax someone's car
- Assist an elderly or disabled person with errands
- Paint a room with or for someone
- Provide rides for someone who can't drive
- Help clean out a cluttered room
- General housecleaning
- Respite break for anyone who is a caretaker
- Volunteer with someone for a cause of their choice

Non-food ideas like those in this chapter do much more than sidestep the problem of overusing food. They make us more active participants in our own lives and relationships. They put us in greater touch with ourselves and with those we care about. They make life more interesting, meaningful, and satisfying. And they work all of this magic while improving our health rather than undermining it.

Chapter 31
Moving as if Your Life Depends on It

In Chapter 4, we looked at how sedentary living compromises quality of life both psychologically and physically. It intensifies any struggles you may have with self-control around food, along with increasing your vulnerability to numerous chronic diseases. While simply sitting less will improve your situation considerably, purposefully incorporating more physical activity will take you even further.

But how do you embrace that when your emotional brain is so resistant to the idea of moving on purpose for no apparent reason? Remember the source of that resistance: the emotional brain sees nothing but up-front effort without immediate payoff when it considers intentional physical activity (exercise). The solution is to pursue that activity in a way that provides some immediate benefits to your emotional brain, enabling you to accrue the longer-lasting emotional and physical benefits that will come as a result of staying the course.

Show Your Emotional Brain a Good Time
There are several ways to make exercise more immediately rewarding for your emotional brain. You've probably seen all of them in use or have even used them yourself without realizing why they make the difference that they do.

Music

You probably know the experience of hearing music that makes you want to jump up and dance. Many of us complain that we don't have as much time for enjoying music as we'd like, so what could be better than exercising to music that you love, which happens to make you want to move anyway?

The more the music makes you feel like dancing, the better. The more closely its speed matches the cadence of your movement, the better, because properly synchronized music can make exercise feel so much easier that it's like getting a power-assist. Fortunately, it's never been easier to create a file of customized exercise music that suits your tastes and which is exactly the right speed for what you want to do.

How do you determine the right speed? Simple. Test a few of your favorite songs by playing them as you perform the activity you have in mind. Some songs will be nowhere near the speed you need, while some will be a bit too zippy and others will drag a little too much. Hopefully, you'll find some that hit the sweet spot and your body will just fall into the rhythm as it moves.

Once you've identified a song that's just right, determine its speed with a BPM (beats per minute) analyzer—available online or as an app—or by counting the beats for 15 seconds and then multiplying by four. You now have that song's speed and in this case, you know your own personal magic speed for that particular exercise. Now it's a simple matter of going through your collection looking for other songs in the same general speed category.

Once you've identified a number of songs that you'd like to use for exercise, you can use sound editing software (available free online) to tweak the speed of any that aren't quite right, altering them so that they're just the way you want them. This can be done without distorting the sound in any way, so you needn't worry about your favorite singer beginning to sound like a chipmunk, for example.

However, you know your music very well and will likely find that if you change its speed beyond a certain point, it just won't seem right. My personal experience is that many songs can be pushed as much as four or even five percent faster or slower without violating the integrity of the music so much that it just feels *wrong*. The ability to change song speed by this small amount is likely to make a *lot* more of your music appropriate for exercising. This is excellent for your emotional brain, because it will get to be entertained by music that it likes while you exercise, and it won't get bored if you have a really long playlist that takes you weeks to get through, one workout at a time.

Don't despair if there is music you'd like to use that is *way* too fast or slow. If it's fast enough, you might be able to use it by moving to every other beat. If it's slow enough, you can move to it in double-time. Anything that works is fair game, as long as you end up liking the end result.

But what about those times when music isn't an option, like when you're walking or cycling around traffic, or simply don't have your player with you? Actually, you're *never* without your music because it's all right there in your memory, all the time. It might be less satisfying to hear the music in your thoughts than to hear it with your ears, but even in your head, music will still provide a boost to anything you're doing. And the great thing about the music in your head is that it's always the perfect speed.

Ideally, music will make exercise more enjoyable for you but for some people, nothing helps; they just hate exercising no matter what. If you are among them, music can still come to your rescue, but in a different way. Given that you need a certain amount of exercise no matter how you feel about it, music can make it more tolerable.

You can use music as an escape by focusing on it very purposefully, leaving your body to go through the necessary motions of exercise while your mind is elsewhere. In this case, the speed of the music won't matter much compared to its ability to simply take you away. When it does, the time will pass more easily for you while your body gets what it needs, and you'll get to enjoy better health and a greater sense of overall wellbeing as a result.

Companionship

Companionship is another way to make exercise more attractive to your emotional brain. In addition to improving your experience of exercise, it might also strengthen a relationship or two. After all, you and your companion(s) will be spending more time together, communicating more, supporting each other while enjoying a sense of shared purpose, and enjoying a wider range of activities together.

As mentioned previously, this is less helpful if it's framed in terms of mutual accountability rather than as companionship to be enjoyed in the context of a shared interest; many people use their obligation to a friend as a way to force their own hand on getting the exercise done.

It's a more positive and inviting approach if you focus instead on looking forward to spending time with someone you enjoy, with the understanding that exercising is what you will do together—your emotional brain will like it a lot better that way. If you're not thrilled about the idea of going for a walk on a particular day, for example, you can still look forward to catching up with a good friend while you happen to be moving. If the two of you decide to make a game of it or even enjoy some friendly competition, so much the better.

One potential drawback to this strategy is the risk of becoming overly dependent on your friend's participation as an incentive to keep moving. It often happens that when friends have paired up for this purpose and one drops out, the other stops exercising soon after. For this reason, I strongly recommend that you pursue your own independent exercise on the other days of the week. You need to be physically active that often anyway, and if you're already accustomed to working out on your own part of the time, you'll be less inclined to quit if it happens that someday, your friend is no longer joining you.

Fun Stuff

Another way to improve the experience of exercise for your emotional brain is to find ways to do it that have authentic emotional appeal: activities that are fun, interesting, or challenging. If you enjoy an activity for its own sake, you get the exercise for free.

Many people reject the notion of exercise, for example, but light right up at the idea of alternatives like dancing, going for a walk in the woods, riding a bicycle, or participating in team sports. When energetic movement is the by-product of something you enjoy doing anyway, your body and your emotional brain both win.

It's even better if you can identify a few different activities of interest, because then you're likely to have options for all seasons, both indoors and out. Weather conditions need never prevent you from having a chance to move, and you won't get bored because you'll have a variety of options at your disposal.

If this approach interests you but you have no idea what you might enjoy doing, one way to get ideas is to go to a large sporting goods store. Make a point of walking every aisle in the place, just looking at everything that's there. As you survey all the various bits of gear and clothing, you'll probably get some ideas, like, *Oh, right, skating—I hadn't thought of that and it might be fun.* You might be prompted to remember when you used to enjoy playing ball or tossing a Frisbee around. Perhaps your interest will be piqued by something you've never tried before, like yoga or kickboxing. There's no telling what might inspire you until you go and see what's there.

You can also check your local community center or Department of Parks and Recreation. If your neighborhood doesn't have recreational facilities, you might be able to find a nearby community that does; many cities and municipalities offer a wealth of organized activities for adults that can get you playing and moving again.

It's worth checking any nearby YMCA or YWCA facilities, as well as other health clubs and fitness centers—you can't know what they offer if you don't ask. Take a look at the class listings for your local community college; even if you don't see a class you want to take, you'll see more ideas for things to consider doing on your own. Finally, have a look at online resources like Meetup.com (www.meetup.com) to learn about informal, activity-oriented groups that may be available somewhere near you.

It doesn't matter how you exercise, it only matters that you *do* exercise. You will be amazed at how much better life feels when you do.

Segment Your Workouts

You segment your workout when you think of it not as a full, continuous event, but rather as a series of much smaller events that happen to be strung together.

Smaller events are advantageous because they are a better fit for the short attention span of the emotional brain. Even better, they create numerous reward points within any given workout, since the completion of each segment is a moment of achievement. Your emotional brain therefore gets payoffs throughout the process rather than having to wait until the very end to have something to feel good about.

Strength training (done with weights or other forms of resistance) is naturally segmented since it involves doing a wide variety of individual exercises for a limited number of repetitions each. Each individual exercise becomes a segment; a 45-minute workout could easily have 40 or more segments, each lasting just a minute or so. Your emotional brain only has to deal with a minute or so at a time and at the end of each one, there's a nice little shot of accomplishment to carry you along to the next.

Aerobic forms of exercise usually lack the obvious segmentation of strength training but readily lend themselves to perceptual segments, nonetheless. If you walk, jog, or cycle, you'll notice certain landmarks that show you're a quarter of the way, a third of the way, halfway, or simply on your way back.

Timed workouts have natural milestones at each five- or ten-minute mark. Each milestone—whatever it is—lets you know that you're getting there, in increments that feel meaningful. Whether you value milestones because they help you appreciate what you've accomplished or because they reassure you that this won't last forever, it feels good each time you reach one.

Segmenting is always a good idea, but it's especially useful on the days when you're having trouble keeping yourself going. Those are the days when you'll be segmenting on the fly, using smaller increments than usual. For example, let's say you like to use a machine (elliptical, stepper, skier, treadmill, bike, etc.) for your exercise, and you like to listen to music while you do it. On this particular day though, you're not feeling the love for the process. You're so anxious to get it over with that you're thinking about bailing out early.

Some minutes in, you decide you might just stick it out until the end of the song that's currently playing, then quit. The song ends, and you notice that if you just keep going for a few more seconds, you'll hit an even minute mark on your timer. When you get to that, you notice the next mile mark isn't too far off, so you might as well keep going until you get that much done.

By the time you get to that mile mark, a song you really love has begun; you enjoy moving to it so much that you're good to go for another four minutes or so. By the time the song ends, you've gotten close to the length of workout that you'd initially planned anyway. You might then decide to just go ahead and finish it, never having felt burdened at any point along the way since you were only committing to a few moments at a time.

You can also segment on the fly while walking, jogging, or cycling. If you're on the road or path and are thinking about cutting it short for the day, just make a goal of getting to a particular landmark first: a certain stop sign, park bench, or distinctive tree, for example. Once you've made it to that marker, you might feel okay about adding another segment, proceeding on to the next distinctive feature you can see or which you happen to know is a bit further along.

Keep adding one short segment at a time until your emotional brain is unwilling to add any more, then turn around or loop back to your starting point. By the time you're done, you will have multiplied the benefit from each added segment due to having a longer return trip. The extra distance won't feel like it matters much on the way back, however, because by then, you're in wrap-up mode and highly motivated to get back to your starting point. You'll cover more ground than you otherwise would have, without ever feeling like you were doing more than you could tolerate.

Such is the power of segmenting. What starts out feeling like just too much can be whittled down into little pieces that feel acceptable. The victory of sticking with a workout on a day like this is even sweeter than it is the rest of the time, because it's even more of an accomplishment.

Segmenting is also an excellent way to get yourself going on those days when you're seriously tempted just to skip it altogether. If you don't feel like doing anything, just do two minutes' worth to start. You can do anything for two minutes, right? If you hate it after two minutes, go ahead and quit, because having an exercise experience that you hate is going to be counterproductive anyway. If you discover that it doesn't seem so bad after all, you can go for two more minutes, and so on. You might be amazed at how much you can get done this way.

Take Advantage of Your Ability to Choose

As noted in Chapter 4, we've spent the past century busily engineering the physical activity out of our lives, and have actually eliminated more of it than we could afford to lose. Now, very few of us move enough to protect and maintain our health.

There were good reasons for many of the changes we made at the time, however. We improved basic chores of life that were hard, dirty, dangerous, boring, or some unfortunate combination thereof—think about doing laundry or digging ditches without any mechanical assistance, for example. Much of the work we did away with was simply burdensome, and we'd only been doing it because there was no choice. Many of the changes we made would actually have resulted in a net improvement to public health if only we'd maintained an adequate level of physical activity in some other way.

While we created the unintended consequence of overly sedentary living, we also created an unprecedented opportunity. We now have the freedom to *choose* what we do in order to maintain the level of physical activity that we need.

Given that maintaining good health requires us to move to some degree whether we feel like it or not, it's remarkable that we get to do so in ways that are tailored to our needs and preferences, scheduled at our greatest convenience. While many of our forebears had no choice but to engage in tiring and difficult manual labor for most of their lives, we can get the exercise we need by doing things like walking in a park, playing sports, or dancing if we want to.

It will probably help to remind your emotional brain of that from time to time.

Affordable Indoor and Outdoor Options

Many of my clients seem to assume that in order to be more physically active, they will have to join a fitness club. They worry about obligating themselves to a lengthy and pricy membership contract (if they can afford it at all), especially with the risk that they'll ultimately join the legions of those who have signed up, committed the money, and then watched it all go to waste anyway.

The only people who really *need* fitness clubs are those who lack practical access to other opportunities, or who have medical issues that require the use of specialized facilities. Some people prefer clubs because they like having a wide variety of exercise options in one location, as well as the availability of on-site personal coaching and group classes. If none of that applies to you, however, it's easy, far cheaper, and more convenient to work out on your own.

Indoor Exercise

Strength training is most often an indoor activity and can be accomplished in a surprising variety of ways, beginning with those that cost nothing at all. Bodyweight exercises, for example—like push-ups, squats, and triceps dips—use your own weight as the source of resistance that develops your muscles. There are dozens of bodyweight exercises to choose from, which you can easily research online.

If you like working with equipment, many additional exercises can be performed with simple hand weights, resistance bands, or low-cost suspension trainers. If you go with weights, you might find that you can get by with just a few pairs at the specific weights that you need rather than investing in a full set. If so, you could buy all the weights you'll ever need for the rest of your life for less than $100. An even more economical alternative, though less favorable from an ergonomics standpoint, is to make your own weights by filling common household containers (plastic jars, jugs with handles) with water, sand, or pennies.

If you prefer to do your strength workouts on a machine, many such machines are available for home use, though they can be pricy and take up a lot of floor space. If you want to go that route, it's a good idea to do a trial run on similar equipment at a store or fitness center first, to assure that you like it enough to invest in one of your own.

Once you've done that, you'll get the best value by watching the market for used equipment. There are generally plenty of good machines for sale, often barely used and sometimes at a steep discount. If you don't see any ads for the equipment you seek, it's always worth placing a "wanted" ad of your own; you never know who might see it and pounce on the opportunity to trade a neglected machine for cash.

Getting good, used equipment cheap is a far better idea than getting new equipment that is inexpensive because it is cheaply made. Bargain equipment tends to have poor ergonomics and construction, making it uncomfortable to use and even potentially unsafe. Such equipment is also prone to premature breakdown, so the money you save up front might end up being wasted altogether.

Strength training is safer, more effective, and more enjoyable if you do it correctly. Proper form is very important because it ensures the correct use of the muscles while minimizing the risk of injury. The easiest way to learn proper form is by watching someone who has it, and who can teach you. This could easily be a fitness-oriented friend, but since few of us have those, the next most obvious choice is an accredited personal trainer (look for ACSM, NETA, or AFAA certifications[1]).

Fortunately, we all have more free access to personal trainers than ever before, via Internet videos. As long as you ensure that you use videos only from industry professionals, you can get very detailed and helpful instruction on every exercise you can imagine, plus quite a few that you'd *never* imagine.

If you have the wherewithal, hiring a personal trainer on a limited basis is an excellent way to get the necessary instruction; there's nothing like real-time feedback from an expert to get you on the right track. For as little as $400-$500, you can get all the information you need to keep working out effectively on your own for a lifetime.

Strength training can be about more than conditioning your muscles, however. Yoga, tai chi, and Pilates are all forms of strength training that include a meditative component while also promoting greater physical flexibility and balance. As such, each offers significant benefits in terms of stress management and relaxation, in addition to fitness. Your best bet, if you have the option, is to get your initial instruction from a trainer with certification specific to the form of movement you have chosen. This will give you a stronger base of general understanding and technique for going on to work independently with DVDs, books, or other resources if you'd like.

Indoor options for aerobic exercise are plentiful as well. As with strength training, many machines have been developed for this purpose and all the same general issues apply. They can be expensive and take up a lot of space; it's good to confirm that you like the exercise before you buy the machine; machines are widely available at nice discounts on the used-equipment market; and quality used ones are a better deal than cheaply made new ones.

Most machines built for aerobic exercise are more complex than those built for strength training, so they are more likely to require occasional maintenance or repair.

No worries if an aerobic machine does not fit well in your life, because you have many other ways to get aerobic activity indoors as well: exercise DVDs, interactive games you can play on your TV, and workouts that are streamed online. Or you can skip all of that and just dance energetically to your favorite music.

Outdoor Exercise

Outdoor activity is wonderfully rejuvenating. It gives you a change of scenery, some fresh air, at least the possibility of sunlight, and some options that are refreshingly different from those activities that you do indoors. Time outdoors is especially well advised if you're trying to stave off or come back from a bout of depression. Many outdoor activities exist, but walking, jogging, and bicycling are by far the most popular.

Walking can probably be done for free with shoes that you already own. If you want to step it up and do some jogging, it might improve your comfort to buy some shoes that have been designed for it. If you notice any pain while walking or jogging, don't ignore it—there might be a problem with your technique or with the fit of your shoes that could eventually result in injury. You can get a consultation on both at many sporting goods stores, often at no charge.

Bicycling is a fun and invigorating option, provided you have somewhere to do it safely. Many people already have a long-neglected bike stuffed away in a corner somewhere, or know someone who does. If you're one of them, this is another way to get started for free or at worst, for a few dollars spent toward whatever maintenance might be necessary to ensure that the bike is fully functional and safe.

If you're cautiously interested in bicycling but don't own one and aren't sure whether you want to make the investment, you might be able to rent one at a nearby park or bike trail. Whether you rent or buy, make sure the seat is adjusted properly for the length of your legs. Casual riders often ride with the seat too low, which puts unnecessary stress on their knees and results in a less enjoyable ride. Any experienced cyclist or bike shop technician can show you the proper adjustment in just a minute or two.

If you do decide to buy a bicycle, keep in mind the same considerations that you do with the purchase of any exercise equipment. Cheaply made bikes are usually not a good deal in the end, and high-quality used bikes are often available at a great price. Occasional safety inspections and minor maintenance will keep any bike on the road for many years; expenses are minimal after the initial purchase.

A Special Note to Homeowners

If you're a homeowner (and therefore probably also a car owner), the most affordable exercise options of all start with the basic necessities of maintaining your property. Many of us farm this work out to others as soon as we can afford to, believing we can make better use of the time in other ways.

Whether it's hiring someone to clean the house, using a car wash, or contracting for lawn maintenance or snow removal services, many of us now pay for the ability to avoid physical tasks which would actually be good exercise if we did them ourselves. Many of us consider such tasks to be undesirable when the reality is that if you are healthy enough to do them safely, they are potentially rewarding in several ways.

They provide the opportunity for physical activity that is productive above and beyond the benefit of providing needed exercise. This is rewarding because it feels good to be productive. It feels good to accomplish something tangible with your time and energy, like creating a tidier home, a neatly trimmed lawn, or a newly cleaned car.

Experiences like this are uniquely grounding and good for overall mental health. As our lives become increasingly technology-based, it behooves us to choose to preserve and maintain such experiences whenever we can.

Segmenting is a great tool when it comes to physical tasks that might feel daunting or undesirable if viewed in their entirety. This can take the form of cleaning a room one area at a time, raking your yard by sections, or waxing your car from one body panel to the next rather than thinking of it as a whole unit.

When you do this, you are effectively focusing on several small tasks—one at a time, done in sequence—rather than trying to take on a big, intimidating project all at once. This will feel better, thus fueling greater motivation. Because you'll be focusing on small tasks rather than trying to rush through a bigger one, you might even do higher quality work.

Many of our labor-saving devices come into play when it comes to home maintenance, and one of your options is to choose your use of them based on how much exercise you want out of your work.

Just because your lawnmower is self-propelled, for example, doesn't mean you always have to use it that way—anytime you want more of a workout, you can choose to push it more of the time on your own. Consider using a rake or broom instead of a leaf blower. If a snowfall is light enough for you to shovel it safely, consider doing at least part of the job—depending on how much exercise you want—that way instead of using the snow blower or paying someone else to take care of it.

You don't have to do any of these things, of course, but if you want to build more exercise into your days, these are some easy ways to do it. And then you get to stand back and admire your work afterward, feeling tired in a good way.

There are worse things.

Move Enough to Create the Life You Want
Of course, the big question is how much general movement and active exercise is the right amount? The general movement part of that question is pretty easy—move as much as you reasonably can. Some ideas:

- Get up often, walking around and stretching a little whenever you have the opportunity. Personally, I try to sit for no longer than 20-30 minutes at a time when I'm planted in front of a computer, for instance.

- If you can't walk anywhere, just walk in place for a moment, preferably with exaggerated high-knee strides that give your leg muscles more of a wake-up call.

- Move more in general by fidgeting on purpose, especially with your legs, since your lower body moves even less than your upper body does when you sit for prolonged periods.

- Be purposely inefficient, making separate trips to other rooms each time you need something rather than batching tasks.

- Stand instead of sitting whenever possible, such as when you're on the phone or even for short periods of time while watching TV. Shift back and forth from one foot to the other as you stand; better yet, lift each foot off the floor a little each time you shift your weight. You might even notice this to be somewhat soothing and pleasant, by the way.

The proper amount of active exercise is less clearly defined, despite the determined efforts of many to do so. The CDC makes a general recommendation of 150 minutes per week of "moderate-intensity aerobic activity" like brisk walking, along with two sessions (length and intensity not specified) of strength training that involves all of the major muscle groups.

The CDC goes on to define several levels of aerobic intensity and provides examples of activities that fit each one.[2] They also offer several schedules of activity at varying combinations of duration and intensity so that you can pick and choose based on what forms of exercise you prefer.

Using 150 minutes per week of moderate aerobic activity as an example, you can accomplish this with five half-hour sessions over the course of a week. Or you can arrange it any other way that you like, as long as you make sure you get at least ten continuous minutes of activity each time you exercise (in order to achieve aerobic benefit). If you do the two strength workouts that are also recommended, that will probably take an additional hour or two of time overall, depending on how comprehensive a workout you choose.

The findings of the National Weight Control Registry (NWCR) are an additional source of information for you to consider. The NWCR has been in operation since 1994, tracking the behavior of thousands of people who have maintained a minimum weight loss of 30 pounds for a year or more.

In reality, the members as a group are far more successful than that, maintaining an average loss of 66 pounds for an average of 5.5 years. Among the relevant statistics, you will find that 98% of them have changed their eating behavior and 94% of them have increased their physical activity, with walking being the activity most often chosen.[3]

When it comes to general movement, it appears that NWCR members may be less sedentary than the general population since 62% of them watch less than ten hours of TV per week. Other forms of screen time are not tracked, however, since the research—which is ongoing—was initially set up in 1994 before most of our current electronic devices were in use. The message is loud and clear on intentional exercise though, as 90% of these people exercise for an average of one hour per day.

NWCR members, by definition, have lost significant amounts of weight. While the average maintained loss is 66 pounds, the *maximum* maintained loss is 300 pounds. It is reasonable to assume that some

NWCR members are living with metabolic changes dating back to their days of obesity, and now need to exercise more than they otherwise would have to in order to maintain a given weight (Chapter 18). For that reason, their needs are probably somewhat different from those of people at the same current weight who have never been obese.

Combining the CDC recommendations and the NWCR research, it appears that the average person, in addition to building much more incidental movement into his or her life, will find the ideal level of exercise somewhere in the range of four to seven hours per week, or an average of 35 to 60 minutes per day, depending on individual need. As it happens, this tracks well with what I have observed for years among the healthiest people I know.

Where *you* fit within these ranges will be a function of many factors, including your genetic heritage, your general health, your weight history, your life circumstances, your typical stress level, and the quality of your diet. Suffice to say that with so many variables in play, it is virtually impossible to calculate the exact requirements for any one individual.

It will be up to you to experiment until you learn what it takes to feel the way you want to feel and to maximize the life quality that is available to you. As always, it's a good idea to consult with your doctor to assure that everything you're doing—especially if you're new to this whole fitness thing—is sensible and safe.

Part Five

Eating with Dignity and Enjoyment for Life

Chapter 32
Eating to Live

Eating to live is the Holy Grail for those who feel enslaved by their compulsion to overeat. It's actually pretty simple, involving basic practices that are effective, rewarding, and empowering. Together, they help you to maintain your focus and get better at bypassing those old neural superhighways in favor of new ones that will serve you better.

First, Do a Reality Check

It's important to keep our current reality in perspective, because it can look like an overwhelming amount of bad news. The problems of processed foods are increasingly well-known but there are numerous concerns about our whole foods as well. These include breaches in food safety, overexposure to agricultural chemicals and other environmental contaminants, the unknown impact of genetic modification, unsustainable land management practices, and inhumane conditions for food animals and food workers alike.

You could easily look at all of this and conclude that it's hopeless, that there are too many problems and that it's not possible to cobble together a healthful, safe, and satisfying diet out of this mess. If you focus too much on all the troubling news, you'll miss the many opportunities you have to make the best of what is available to you.

Life on this planet has always been about trying to survive, and survival has always been about overcoming challenges. The challenges faced by humanity in the modern world are historically unique in some ways, but they're hardly insurmountable. In fact, we share some interesting parallels with our forebears despite the very different world in which we live.

For example, our ancestors were at risk of malnourishment because they often couldn't get enough food. We are at risk of malnourishment because we often don't get enough *food* either. Many of our readily available edibles do not actually support survival.

The acquisition of food was a hazardous venture for our ancestors; many of them died due to physical injuries sustained in the process of trying to keep themselves fed. The acquisition of food is hazardous in a different way today; many of us are dying due to *physiological* injuries sustained in the process of trying to keep ourselves fed.

The trappings of modern life can make it easy to forget that the laws of survival still apply to us, but they do. Basic survival has always been about food and security for yourself and your loved ones, and it has always been challenging in one way or another. It's challenging in an unexpected way now, but other than that, it's the same story it has always been.

So, we're here now and we have today's challenges to tackle; we just need to get better at sidestepping the tempting hazards and doing the best we can with the flawed supply of food that we have. At least we *have* food, for the most part.

And we rarely risk being attacked by wildlife or having a terrible accident while getting breakfast, so *that's* good. On, then, to the mechanics of living more successfully with food in the modern world.

Keep a Safe Home Base

One definition of home is "relaxed and at ease, comfortable."[1] Ideally, home is our sanctuary, our quiet refuge from the challenges and demands of the outside world; it's where we can fully relax.

The reality is that many homes fail this definition for a variety of reasons beyond the scope of this book, including relational problems, financial stress, and even basic personal safety. It's important for anyone to make home a place where you can relax more of the time when it comes to food, but all the more so if your home is otherwise a source of stress in your life.

If you've had problems with overeating, a home that is safe and relaxing with food is a home where you don't have to fight to maintain self-control. This doesn't mean that you relax your way right into a regrettable binge once you get there. It means that bingeing is not a high risk because there are no foods present which are known to trigger you that way.

A safe home is stocked with plenty of enjoyable food that meets all of your needs, and excludes foods that are likely to cause you to lose control. Even better, a safe home is one in which nobody gets pressured to eat and nobody gets teased for wanting to take good care of themselves. A safe home is an easy place to relax, recharge, stay healthy, and feel strong.

If you are an adult running your own household, your home may be the only place in which you have the power to create such an environment. If you do, your time at home will be a time of ease, allowing you to conserve your limited stores of willpower for the challenges of the outer world. If you don't, your home will mirror the food problems of the outer world, leaving you nowhere to hide, nowhere to rest, and with no hope for change. If you can't fully rest and relax around food at home, where can you ever do it?

If you make your home safe, you're more likely to find the determination to keep *yourself* safer when you're in other environments as well. Having discovered how nice it is to be able to relax and enjoy food calmly at home, you'll become more aware of how stressful it actually is elsewhere, and perhaps less willing to subject yourself to it when you don't have to. It will become easier to make the choices that reduce your risk when you discover that you're actually much happier that way.

Whether or not they appreciate it, a home that is safe in this way is also of great benefit to all others who live there. Even if no one else in the home thinks or cares about it, it will be easier for them to be healthier anyway.

If you have kids, they'll probably leave this valuable experience behind for a time when they launch and start experimenting with how to set up their own lives, but the lesson-by-example will be there for them in the future if and when they're ready. Thanks to you, they'll at least know that living this way is possible. They'll see how it's done, and they'll see how much healthier and more able you are than the parents of most of their friends. It's the best that you can do.

Design New Patterns That You Fully Enjoy

Using the information in this book, you can develop practices with food and general self-care that create *only* good emotional and physical outcomes. You can enjoy your eating, feel empowered by your day-to-day practices, enjoy improving health, and live free of both resentment and regret. This is the path to maximizing both quality of life and long-term success with food. Don't settle for less.

If your practices don't accomplish this for you or if they feel burdensome to maintain, it simply means that your system needs more refinement. The answers exist, but you'll only find them if you refuse to continue living without them.

Eat in Response to Hunger

Ideally, the only reason you would ever eat would be when you were physiologically hungry. Beyond that, you consume calories that your body doesn't need and can't use. Realistically, you will sometimes eat for other reasons, but it's important to remember that each time you do, you begin to create an energy imbalance (more calories going in than are getting used) which will result in fat storage. Therefore, it's important to be highly selective about when you eat for reasons other than hunger, and to be very aware of how much you eat at those times.

The first order of business then, if you're considering eating something, is to assess whether you're actually hungry. Is your body asking for food, or do you just want to eat because you like to eat?

Some people notice hunger through clear physical sensations like a feeling of emptiness or growling in the stomach, while others notice it in more subtle ways like becoming shaky, lightheaded, irritable, or less able to think clearly. Short of experiencing your particular signs, whatever they are, your body doesn't need food yet.

If you conclude that you'd really like to eat and that it isn't because your body is asking for food, the next thing to assess is why. Is it because you're stressed, bored, or upset about something? Are you looking for a way to take an emotional break? Do you just want something to do? Are you feeling antsy and looking for a way to focus your energy?

If you can identify the real reason you want to eat, then you can try addressing the need with a non-food strategy (Chapter 24) that is likely to help you feel better than food could anyway.

There are two reasons that it's always best to use physiological hunger as your cue to eat. First and foremost, unless your systems of hunger regulation have been disrupted (which is uncommon, but can happen), it means your body is ready for food. Hunger is your natural green light that it's a valid time to eat. Second—and of far greater interest to your emotional brain—is that when you're actually hungry, food tastes its very best. You will never get more flavor from each calorie than when you are legitimately hungry before beginning to eat.

To be clear though, mindfulness about hunger means that you eat when you are *hungry*, rather than waiting until you are starving. You might occasionally end up overly hungry due to unexpected circumstances, but it happens more often due to inattentiveness, poor planning, or both.

Excessive hunger is to be avoided for three compelling reasons. First, feeling painfully hungry means that you are likely to shovel down anything you can get your hands on as soon as you get the opportunity. Second, you'll be eating with such speed and urgency that you won't be able to notice much of the sensory reward of the food, so you'll probably compensate for the missed reward by shoveling in more. Third and perhaps most devastating, the hunger mechanism might not shut down after you've consumed a reasonable amount of food—or even after you've consumed a *lot* of food.

When the body gets into a crisis of deep hunger, the normal mechanisms of self-regulation can temporarily fail, resulting in an ongoing drive to keep eating even after a large amount of food has already been consumed. This state can induce a damaging binge that is frightening in terms of sheer, extended loss of control. It is to be avoided at all costs.

The final component of eating in response to hunger is that you stop eating once your hunger is satisfied. Not when you are stuffed, but when there is no longer any trace of hunger. If you feel pleasantly full in a way that doesn't make your clothing fit differently, you've nailed it. If you are at all uncomfortable or your clothing has gotten tight, you've probably overeaten, because proportional eating will not create those problems.

The sense of physical satiety can take 15-20 minutes to register fully. It's a good idea to make a point of stopping a little sooner than you really want to, because you'll continue to feel more of the effects of your meal in the minutes that follow. The vast majority of the time, you'll end up being glad you quit "early," because you'll find out after the fact that it was actually the right time (or even a bit late). It's important to pay attention to how this works for you so that over time, you gradually get better at gauging when to stop.

Fortunately, there may be another way to gauge when it's time to stop eating, and it happens in real time rather than on a delayed basis. As mentioned above, food tastes the very best when you're physically hungry. Many people have noticed that as their hunger is satisfied over the course of a meal, the flavor hit of the food becomes less pronounced. If you're paying close attention, you might notice that the flavor gradually shifts from being great, to really good, to merely good, depending on much of it you eat.

When the food no longer tastes exceptional, that's usually about the right time to stop. Try stopping at that point, and then note your physical fullness 20 minutes later to see how the two correlate. With practice, you'll get better at using the two signs together to perfect your timing.

By the way, think about that idea of the food tasting less wonderful as you continue to eat it. If you stop eating as the flavor becomes less impressive, it will taste wonderful all over again if you save the rest for another time when you're hungry. Win-win.

Eat Mindfully

You can't possibly control something when you don't know that it's happening, so you can't control your eating if you aren't paying attention when you do it. Eating more mindfully is critical to creating the relationship with food that you want.

Eating mindfully is actually a lovely thing. It means taking time to slow down, *sit* down, and really notice your food when you eat. It does *not* mean purposely chewing each bite dozens of times, turning it into a disgusting mess in your mouth before you swallow.

What it *does* mean is noticing one wonderful bite at a time, taking care to miss none of the enjoyment before you swallow. Try to taste and feel all of it before it goes, not starting the next bite until you've fully enjoyed the previous one.

It helps a lot to take smaller bites, simply because less of the food will escape untasted by the time you swallow. The goal is to eat more slowly and with greater attention in order to maximize your enjoyment; the fact that it will reduce your caloric intake is a handy bonus.

When you maximize your enjoyment of each bite, you may find that it takes fewer bites to satisfy you. By eating more slowly, you give your body more time to let you know when it's had enough. By paying more attention, you are able to notice which foods live up to your expectations and which foods are actually not as good as you've been giving them credit for; you may ultimately decide that some foods are no longer worthy of space in your life.

Eating mindfully means focusing your attention on your food, so you need to minimize eating while splitting your attention with other things like reading, driving, or watching any screen. When circumstances require you to divide your attention, remain aware that this decreases both your self-control and your enjoyment of the food. It's a lose-lose proposition to be avoided whenever possible.

Eat Real Food
Real food with minimal processing is the key to both good health and comfortable self-control. As Dr. David Kessler noted in his brilliant book, *The End of Overeating*, "The enduring ability to eat differently depends on coming to see these (processed) foods as enemies, not friends." Some processed foods can come in handy in limited circumstances but for the most part, you need to stick to real food.

Whenever you choose a manufactured food, you need to read the label. Don't pay much attention to the splashy labels on the front, with their healthy-sounding buzzwords that often mean nothing. Those are meant to entice, not to inform. Look elsewhere on the package for the nutritional information and the list of ingredients. Look for products that have more fiber, more protein, less sodium, and less sugar than their shelf mates, and which are composed of ingredients that you understand.

Beware the "healthy" versions of sweet treats and salty snacks that are otherwise notorious for their lack of nutrition. They might indeed be less damaging than their counterparts, but they often turn out simply to be damaging in a different way, reformulated based on being more marketable rather than more nutritious. In any event, they are unlikely to *support* health. To make unfortunate use of a food-related adage, there is no free lunch. If it sounds too good to be true, it almost certainly is.

Just stick with real food (Chapters 3 and 14) so that you don't have to worry about any of that, and make sure you stay well stocked with it, too. Don't ever leave your emotional brain lacking for attractive, easy, nutritious options when the need hits.

If you'd like to transition toward a balanced diet of real food but feel confused about where to start, you have lots of company. Fortunately, it's not that hard to sort out because, remember, quality nutrition is not complicated. If you'd feel better with some guidance, however, consider looking into the Mediterranean diet, widely recommended as a good template for enjoyably eating your way to robust health.[2] You can find lots of helpful introductory information at http://oldwayspt.org/traditional-diets/mediterranean-diet.

Finally, if you have any medical conditions as a result of being overweight or obese, it's a good idea to consult with a Registered Dietician Nutritionist, preferably one who understands disordered eating and integrative medicine. Good resources can be found at www.integrativerd.org and www.SCANdpg.org, professional associations within the Academy of Nutrition & Dietetics, where emphasis is placed not just on nutritional issues, but also on how you relate to food.[3]

Do Most of Your Own Cooking

There are several compelling reasons to prepare your own food much more of the time. One obvious factor is expense, since it's cheaper to do your own cooking than to pay someone else to do it for you. It's certainly fair to pay a premium for the service, but the cumulative impact on your finances can be severe if you often eat food prepared by others, as so many people now do. If expenses are tight or you are accumulating debt, cooking at home is an effective countermeasure.

Some prepared foods that are purchased outside the home might seem like a bargain, but that's usually due to their being based on inexpensive filler ingredients that you wouldn't put in your own food even if you could buy them yourself. Such foods might *seem* economical because they cost less to buy today, but they come at tremendous expense to your future health and quality of life. Money spent on quality food in the present is one of the best investments you can make.

When you cook your own food, you are in control of its nutritional value. You know exactly what's in the food because you put it there. The risk of buying food prepared by others is that even dishes based on whole foods might include shocking amounts of added sodium, sweeteners, and fats. The food is delicious, of course, but again at a cost to your future health that is not obvious in the moment of sensory delight.

Another important point, then, is that doing your own cooking allows you to reduce your exposure to triggering foods dramatically. When you're the cook, you are completely in control of the level of challenge you face. Commercially produced food, on the other hand, is designed specifically to *make* you want to eat and eat and eat ... and then to want to come back many more times to do it all over again. You will simply make it much easier to maintain your self-control if you reduce your exposure to food prepared outside your home.

There's yet another reason to cook your own food which might surprise you, and it has to do with our roots. It's natural to devote a lot of personal attention to the subject of food. It has historically taken a tremendous amount of humanity's time and energy to acquire enough food to survive. That time used to involve searching for the food, hunting it down or gathering it up, bringing it home, preparing it for consumption, and then actually eating it.

That's a *lot* of time, physical effort, and psychological activity dedicated specifically to food. Most of humanity has *had* to focus on food to that degree and much of humanity still does; we're wired for it.

As it is now though, many of us in areas of even moderate population density no longer have to work much at all in order to eat. Whether you're walking in the city or driving in the suburbs, you could easily be within minutes of dozens of options for getting food: fast food places, cafes, conventional restaurants, food trucks, convenience stores, and—to a much lesser degree—grocery stores.

Eating has historically been the smallest part of the food-acquisition process, but now it's almost the whole process! While it's always been natural and necessary to *think* about food a lot of the time, it hasn't been natural to *eat* a lot of the time, especially when it involves the ultra-high-calorie options available to us today.

We still possess a powerful, inborn drive to focus on food and we need to satisfy that drive somehow—we just can't afford to do it exclusively through eating. The logical solution is to increase our involvement with food in other ways, and that means going back to cooking at home.

Provided you don't snack your way through the process, home-cooking gives you outlets for food-related energy and interest that go beyond the act of eating. You get to research recipes, learn about new ingredients, and try new ideas. You get to handle and work with your food as you go through the physical actions of cooking.

You get to be involved, once again, in the *process* of feeding yourself and your family. You get to play with food and be with food in ways that add value rather than taking it away, all while increasing the quality of the food available for yourself and your loved ones.

Taking cooking classes is another way to focus constructively on food, as is tending a home garden. Focus more on the acquisition side of the food equation, and you may find that you have less excess energy looking for an outlet on the consumption side.

Just be careful about tasting as you cook. It's necessary to do this to a limited degree to assure that your creation is on track, but it's easy to overstep, especially if your dish is turning out really well. Tasting can quickly become another form of grazing: little nibbles that, together, add up to be a lot more food than you'd guess. They feel like they don't count, and your emotional brain will certainly tell you they don't count, but they do. It all counts.

When it comes to the final phase of the process—the actual eating—there's another compelling benefit of cooking at home and focusing on whole foods, especially if you are also transitioning toward a more plant-based diet along the way. Such foods have fewer calories than their alternatives.

You're probably accustomed to thinking of lower-calorie foods as a tool for losing weight, but if you've had trouble with overeating, consider this: When food has fewer calories, you get to eat more of it.

This is important because as much as we like tasty foods, we also like the actual behavior of eating. We like it a lot. We like to handle food, play with it in our mouths, swallow it, and feel ourselves getting filled by it. We like all of those physical aspects of the eating experience, independent of what we actually consume.

Lower-calorie foods mean that the behavioral part of the fun lasts a lot longer than it can when you eat higher-calorie foods. Personally, I love huge salads for a meal. Why? Because while I appreciate that they are packed with nutrition, what I *love* is that they take so long to eat.

A well-constructed salad allows me to play with food for as long as 45 minutes, while consuming a fraction of the calories I'd have gotten from wolfing down some fast food thing in just five or ten minutes. The nutritional value and absence of additives is a great bonus, much appreciated by my cortex. My emotional brain is just happy because it gets to play with food for a long time. Win-win.

Create More Food-Free Space in Your Life

Chapter 2 recalled the norms of generations past when food was only acceptable in certain places and at certain times. It wasn't obvious until after we abandoned those patterns, but it was a lot easier to eat within reasonable limits when we had them. Now, we are chronically overexposed to food; it can show up almost anywhere at almost any time, which means we have to deal with it and think about it many times per day.

Research conducted at Cornell University showed that while study participants *thought* they made 15 food-related decisions per day, they actually made well over 200.[4] We wrestle with food-related thoughts a great deal of the time, and much more than we realize. Whether we're aware of the process or not, it is tiring and stressful, as well as presenting the opportunity for many, many food-related mistakes.

This burden would be reduced considerably if only we could escape to some spaces in our lives where food was simply not present. When food is not there and you know it's not going to *be* there, you naturally think about it a lot less.

For a radical example of how this works, think of the last time you were required to fast in preparation for a medical procedure. For a prescribed number of hours, you understood that food would not be an option, probably because you either wanted the results of the medical procedure or simply wanted to get it over with so you wouldn't have to do it again on some other day. Either way, you had no food-related decisions to consider for a set period of time.

During that time, you had no internal chatter about what to do, how much to have, or whether you could stand how you were dealing with food right then. Other than pondering what you'd eat once the procedure was over, you had absolutely no food-related decisions to make for hours on end. For once, the raging internal debate was quiet. You might have been hungry and you might have felt sad about not getting to eat, but you probably had a level of internal peace you seldom get to enjoy.

You can have more of that peace—every day for the rest of your life—and you don't have to fast in order to achieve it (unless you really want to).

How to Create and Use Food-Free Space

Consider the circumstances in which you do most of the eating that troubles you. What if you just decided that you would no longer eat in *those* particular circumstances, reserving your eating for the situations in which it already tends to work out a lot better anyway?

Doing this wouldn't take anything away; it would just rearrange how and when you eat. This would make your life with food much easier and more relaxing, but if you felt some initial resistance to the idea, you could always try it on a limited basis as an experiment. If you didn't like it, you'd simply stop doing it. The experiment would be risk-free.

If you're interested in trying this, the first thing you'll need to do is think about the various physical locations in which you eat. Most people who overeat do so in many places, commonly including most rooms of the home (including decks and porches), motor vehicles, and at their work area when on the job—almost anywhere they ever spend time, basically.

This matters because you naturally have food-related thoughts wherever you're used to eating. If you eat practically everywhere, you'll have to struggle with those thoughts most of the time. Spend more time in places that you don't associate with eating, and you'll have fewer of those thoughts to manage; it's a remarkably easy way to reduce the effort required for maintaining self-control with food.

Don't worry if every physical location you can think of already seems to be heavily associated with eating. This isn't the obstacle it would seem to be because it is surprisingly easy to change. Think about the places where your most destructive eating occurs, and just decide to not eat in *those* places anymore. Ideally, you'll eliminate eating almost everywhere other than one or two areas within your home, one spot at work, and outside locations like restaurants or the homes of friends or family.

If this sounds extreme, that's only because it's different from what you're used to doing. It actually does *nothing* to restrict your ability to eat. It simply causes you to be more thoughtful about it when you do, and to make the minor effort of moving to one of the locations you've designated for eating when the time comes. It rebuilds some structure around the act of eating, a necessary change given that the anywhere/anytime approach has proven to be so damaging.

Once you do this, there will be many times when it crosses your mind to eat, but when you realize you don't care about it enough to bother relocating just so you can do it. Each time this happens, you will effortlessly eliminate some bit of eating that otherwise would have happened for no good reason.

Better yet, you'll get to see that thoughts of eating often aren't all that powerful; it's comforting to discover that some of them are actually fairly easy to ignore if you have any immediate incentive for doing so. Sometimes, your emotional brain gets more reward from staying where it is than it would from going somewhere else just to eat, so you can feel content to let the thought pass. It's pretty great when that happens.

Next, think about the activities that you often pair with eating and consider which of those activities commonly correlate with eating in ways that you later regret. Common culprits are activities performed in the places mentioned previously: watching TV or other screens, reading, local travel, and work, plus any additional activities that are specific to your personal circumstances. Once you've identified the activities most associated with your overeating, you just decide that you will no longer engage in eating while doing them.

You still engage in all of your activities. You still eat when you choose to. You just don't combine them anymore. If you want the activity, stop eating and go do it. If you want to eat, stop the activity and go do it. The result is that you will eat only when you care enough about it to choose it over your other options. You might be surprised to see how often you elect to stick with your activity, again noticing that the urge to eat is not as all-powerful as you've assumed.

When you do choose to eat, you can do it in a mindful and dignified way, keeping your attention on the food until you're done. You'll be noticing how enjoyable the food is rather than shoveling it down mindlessly while paying attention to something else. If the calories are going into your system anyway, you might as well get the maximum enjoyment out of them; mindful eating is the key to doing that.

By the way, one sign of a truly engaging activity is one that you hate to stop even when your stomach is growling with hunger. On those occasions, *do* listen to your stomach and take a meal break, perhaps while noticing how lovely it is to experience a thought like, *Aw, I have to stop so I can eat, and I really don't want to.* It's an exhilarating departure from, *I want to stop eating but I can't.*

Adapting Your Strategies to Meet Specific Needs

No discussion of food-free space can be complete without a warning about all-or-nothing thinking. Let's say you're focusing on eating a more nutritious diet, and you've also decided you'll no longer eat in your car. What do you do on a road trip? You can avoid eating in your car by eating at restaurants along the way ... but it's hard to find anything other than triggering fast-food restaurants on the road. You could take your own nutritious food along so that you're staying out of the restaurants, but now you're eating in your car and you weren't going to do that anymore.

What's the answer when priorities seem to collide? The answer is to stay in the game, keep your eye on what keeps you feeling calm and in control with food, and make the best accommodations that you can.

Personally, I take my own food on the road and eat in the car, which is the only time I ever eat in a car. For a long day trip, I always have to fight the urge to pack food as if I was preparing for a week-long trek into the wilderness. Each time, I gently remind myself that while it feels like a big deal to cover hundreds of miles, I'm actually just sitting totally still for an entire *day* and my caloric needs will be quite modest. Having regained my perspective, I pack enough for a moderate lunch and dinner.

But that's not actually the most important part of my food planning for a road trip. The most important thing I bring along—from my emotional brain's perspective—is the ample supply of dry, low-calorie, high-fiber cereal that I will munch on by hand whenever I want to (another departure from my usual habits), because I know that hours on the road always make me want to eat. Since dry cereal is not at all triggering for me, I munch on it whenever I'm feeling the urge, and just stop once I get tired of it.

Note that I don't try to ignore or power through urges to munch while on the road—I plan ahead to satisfy them harmlessly. Because my nutritional *and* munching needs are being met adequately in the car, I don't have to think about buying anything (including beverages, since I have lots of water in the car) at a rest stop where the selections are so marginal.

These practices have kept me from ever having a regrettable food experience on the road, despite that situation being such an ideal setup for destructive eating. I don't foresee any problems with it in the future either, because I know what works for me and I just stick to it. It might sound boring, but my experience is that it is calming. Calm is good.

Chances are that, like me, you'll establish a basic set of practices that serves you well most of the time, and then find that there are occasional outlier experiences requiring a different set of practices to keep you comfortably in control. Anything that gets you through with composure and lack of regret is the right thing to do. You just need to try different ideas to see what works for you, and then to make sure that you always plan for what you need.

For another example, I had to make some adjustments concerning eating while watching TV, because I was doing an enormous amount of out-of-control eating that way. The simple answer would be to just make TV-watching a food-free activity, but I could easily tell that if I tried to commit to that, I'd have an internal rebellion on my hands and the whole system would collapse.

Therefore, I decided I would eat while watching TV only under limited circumstances. At that time, I decided that I would still watch while eating dinner or while munching on popcorn (air-popped, no oils) if I wanted to. That decision enabled me to easily let go of the eating/TV combination the rest of the time, and to do so with no bad feelings at all. I have since found that as long as it's a real meal eaten in response to physical hunger, I can eat while watching without any loss of self-control, so breakfast and lunch are now included as well.

I haven't eliminated eating while watching TV; that might have been the apparent ideal, but it wouldn't have worked for very long. I have thoroughly eliminated eating *destructively* while watching TV, and that's been good enough to support solid results for a very long time. In service to that, I don't eat triggering foods while watching TV, ever. And I wouldn't want to anyway at this point, because if I'm going to eat something purely for entertainment value, I want to give it my undivided attention so that I don't miss any of it.

I offer my practices not as a template for anyone else to follow—we each need to find our own best way—but as an example of practices that hit all the important goals. They protect the body while remaining acceptable to *and* safe for the emotional brain. As such, they create a satisfying and comfortable way to live, and are easily sustainable for life.

If you want a set of benchmarks to aim for as you develop your own practices, those are about as good as it gets. Rest assured that such practices are not discovered overnight. They come as a result of ongoing experimentation and refinement, so you'll probably find yourself gradually modifying and improving yours for quite some time.

Though it's not strictly necessary to keep notes on the various things that you try and how they work out, you might find it beneficial if you do; memory alone can be an unreliable source of this kind of information over time. Regardless of how you go about it, it's a fascinating project that is well worth your attention.

Cut Portions Back Down to Size
We need to reclaim boundaries around our eating as described above, but we also need to reclaim them when it comes to our notions of portion size. It is common now, for example, to order dinner out and receive an amount of food that could easily stretch to a second or even third meal, yet attempt to consume it in one sitting.

We do it to ourselves at home as well, using large plates and bowls for convenience and then unconsciously loading them up with more food than we realize. And that's when we even portion out our food at all. A great deal of overeating gets done straight from the main supply: the chip bag, the ice cream carton, the brownie pan, the container full of leftovers.

We have become accustomed to quantities of food that make no practical sense at all. This is a tough one for the emotional brain, because there's really nothing to do but somehow throttle back our expectations and get accustomed to smaller portions.

Smaller plates and bowls are an important way to make the transition more comfortably, because we tend to focus on units of consumption rather than on the size of those units. For example, when you eat a bowl of soup, you probably just think of it as "a bowl of soup," rather than focusing much on whether it's a big bowl or a small one.

To understand how you can use this to your advantage, imagine two bowls, side by side, one twice the size of the other. Fill the small one with soup, creating a bowl of soup. Put the exact same amount of soup in the larger bowl, and you have created *half* a bowl of soup.

There's no more soup in the smaller bowl yet it's more satisfying to look at, so you're more likely to feel that the serving is an acceptable size. This perceptual quirk is the reason that smaller dishes are so helpful in portion control. They allow you to eat less without feeling the difference nearly as much.[5]

As you transition your way down to smaller sizes of dinnerware, take time after each meal to notice how your body feels. Twenty minutes after you've eaten, do you still feel physically hungry, are you comfortably satisfied, or do you feel stuffed? Use this information to get better at gauging your portions over time. When in doubt, take a little less than you think you really want just to see how it works out. You might be surprised at how often that ends up being the right amount after all.

You definitely want to avoid the error of taking too much food, for two reasons. First, you'll eat more just because there's more food in front of you.[6] Second, you'll tend to want to eat all of it simply because that's what most of us do—we clean our plates, no matter how much food was on them to start with. The lesson here is to be very, very careful about how much food you allow to end up in front of you because once it's there, you'll feel a strong drive to finish it no matter what.

Second servings call for even greater care. When you're considering a second serving, your body has only just begun to work on what you've eaten already and has not yet been able to send the satiety signal. However, your taste buds are now fully activated and your emotional brain is clamoring for more—lots more.

The most important thing to remember about second servings is that quite often, if you wait a few minutes, you'll find you are already physically satisfied and in need of no additional food after all.

If you are quite sure that you need more to satisfy your physical hunger—remembering your emotional brain will always tell you that you need more, regardless of your physical state—try taking half the amount that you think you really need. Chances are very good that by the time you finish it, you'll find it was actually the perfect amount and you'll be glad that there's nothing left on the plate goading you to keep eating just because it's there.

A final note on portion management is the importance of no longer eating directly from the main supply of any food, like a platter of leftovers, a family-sized tub of yogurt, or a box of crackers. We generally do this with the intention of having just a little bit and then putting the rest away. Many of us do it to avoid the unnecessary dirtying of a dish we'll later need to wash, though some of us do it in the hope that the eating won't count if nobody can tell we did it.

Whatever the motive, if your cortex's plan is to nibble directly from the food until you've had enough, your emotional brain will immediately redefine "enough" as all of the food in front of you. You'll then need to make yourself stop when the easiest thing would be to keep on eating, and chances are you'll eat a lot more than you intended. It's a setup for regret that is easy to avoid.

It's far better to use a plate or bowl to portion out your food, and then put the rest away before you begin to eat. Putting the rest of it away first is important because the second your taste buds activate on the food and your emotional brain gets into higher gear, your judgment and decision-making skills will plummet. If you haven't already put the rest of the food away, you'll probably end up going back for more of it just because it's still right there. You can make your life much easier by clearing the area of unnecessary triggers before you get that first taste.

*　*　*　*　*

Don't worry if the suggestions in this chapter bear little resemblance to your usual practices—that's to be expected. Your usual practices haven't worked well for you, so it's logical that you'll need to do some things differently if you want better outcomes.

Your emotional brain is likely to greet these new patterns with some reluctance each time you practice them, and then to be pleasantly surprised each time when things turn out well after all. And then it will forget and you'll have to gently coax it along all over again to get the same satisfying results the next time. As mentioned previously, this may seem inconvenient but it results in a far happier life than if you don't do it. It's a small price to pay for what you get in return.

Chapter 33
Keeping It Together in Challenging Situations

Having just detailed the ways in which you can set yourself up to have a better relationship with food, we need to talk now about how to cope with the fact that food will still remain challenging at times anyway. It's simply the reality of the world in which we live, so your best bet is to develop some strategies for making the best of it.

Include Treat Foods Only in Life-Affirming Ways

There's room in life for treat foods, but it doesn't take much before they do more harm than good. If you're going to include them, you need to do so very carefully.

Your body can use only so many calories, and treat foods burn through that allotment very quickly. Worse yet, treat foods often replace calories that would have carried essential nutrients with calories that carry unsafe substances. You can't afford to displace many nutrients or to ingest much that is potentially harmful, so treat foods can occupy only a limited space in your world before they start doing damage.

Because treat foods are notoriously triggering to the emotional brain, including them in your system of eating means that you'll have to work harder at maintaining control. You might find this tradeoff completely acceptable—it's just important that you understand you're making it. Because treat foods are so challenging, you need to be very selective about which ones you choose and the circumstances in which you have them.

Careful portioning is more important with treat foods than with anything else we eat because they are so triggering and high in calories. Serving size must be considered carefully, balancing your desire for the food with your desire for the life you want to have—the serving size that will satisfy *both* will probably be a lot smaller than you're used to. Once you've gotten your serving ready and have put away the rest, sit down somewhere comfortable and without distractions, and savor every bite.

You might have a strong desire to go back for more of your treat once you've finished, due to the overstimulation of your taste buds and your emotional brain. This is the way treat foods routinely affect us, so you might as well prepare for it.

It may get you past the moment of temptation if you remind yourself that you selected your initial portion size for very good reasons in the first place. You felt that you could get enjoyment without any unwanted aftereffects, so if you go back for more now you will almost certainly end up regretting it.

Having reminded yourself of that, you might then take a big gulp of water and swish it around in your mouth well before swallowing it. Then take another gulp of water and do the same. What you'll be doing is rinsing the triggering flavor off of your tongue.

When the taste buds stop firing, it's much easier for the emotional brain to calm back down so you can stay in control. Less than five minutes later, you'll probably be over the whole thing, happy to have had the treat and *really* happy to have stopped when you did.

If this sounds like a lot of strategizing for something as simple as a yummy snack, it's because yummy snacks can launch you quickly into the red zone, so you need to approach them with great care. If you're not willing to make this level of effort to eat them safely, your only other reasonable option is to forego them altogether, something few of us are willing to do.

If eating mindfully is important with food in general, it is even more so with treat foods. Treat foods are very high-risk; you can't afford to increase the risk further by eating them with only partial attention. For that reason, I strongly recommend that you have no distractions of any kind when eating a treat food. Just have it in a quiet setting, giving it your full attention so you don't miss any part of the enjoyment, remaining aware of whether you're starting to feel wobbly in your self-control.

A final note about treat foods pertains to a consequence of their caloric density that was alluded to earlier. We like the physical act of eating and we enjoy spending a fair amount of time at it, but high-calorie foods satisfy the body's energy needs long before we've had nearly enough chew time. As a result, you need to keep the serving size of treat foods quite small in order to maximize the total amount of time that you get to spend eating in a given day. Unfortunately, the size of those servings will necessarily shrink further as your metabolic needs decrease over time. This is not great news but it is the reality, so you need to be aware of it.

This isn't to dissuade you from incorporating treat food at a workable level if you wish, but to make you aware of the trade-off to your emotional brain, which likes both the sensory impact of food and the act of eating it. Your challenge is to balance those needs in the way that keeps you the happiest and healthiest, and to understand that you'll need to revisit the calculation from time to time as your age, health, and circumstances change.

Buy Yourself Some Time When You're Having an Urge to Eat
Many people believe that the moment they feel an unwanted food urge, all hope is lost. Believing that loss of control is inevitable anyway, they quickly succumb in the hope of at least ending the internal torment.

As it happens, many of these urges are weaker than you'd guess. A surprising number of them actually can be forgotten completely if you get distracted for a few minutes, whether by coincidence or design. For that reason, it always pays to stall if you can. You'll be much more successful at that if you've previously developed a list of strategies for it, perhaps titled along the lines of *Things to Do Instead*.

It's important to create this list when you're not in the grip of an urge, because you can't think very well about alternatives once your emotional brain has locked onto the idea of food. I have assisted in the construction of many such lists, and recommend the following general parameters:

- The list should consist of at least 25-30 different choices. This may sound like a lot, but with that many to choose from, the chances are good that in any given moment, at least one of them will feel acceptable.

- Each item on the list should be something that you can bring to completion within five to fifteen minutes; your emotional brain is much more willing to agree to a diversion if it doesn't involve a lengthy time commitment. It's okay if some of your selections are activities that you can do for longer if you want to once you've started them, but you must never *commit* yourself to more than the initial maximum of 15 minutes.

- Include some items that you really enjoy, especially those things for which you seldom feel you have the time. If you're on the verge of spending time making a mistake with food, you officially have some time available to take advantage of in some more rewarding way. Common examples include reading for pleasure, playing some music, playing with a pet, doing your nails, messaging or calling a friend, or simply relaxing for a few guilt-free minutes.

- Include little personal and household management tasks that will help you feel lighter and less burdened once you've gotten them out of the way. Common examples include deleting items from email folders, straightening up the kitchen, doing one phase of a load of laundry, dusting or vacuuming a room or two, cleaning out some office files, sorting a pile of mail, doing some shredding, throwing out some old catalogs, selecting a handful of clothing items for donation, or pulling a few weeds.

- Do not include any alternatives that you find flatly unattractive. For example, if the alternative activity is to spend five minutes cleaning the toilet, you might just as well prefer going for the food, so that's not helpful. Unless, of course, you like the idea of getting that task out of the way—in that case, go for it. It's all about what your emotional brain finds acceptable in the moment.

- Get your list in print rather than just brainstorming and hoping you'll remember your good ideas when the time comes. Your problem-solving and strategic ability will be compromised once you start focusing on food, but you'll probably be able to remember that the list exists and go to it for ideas as needed.

  After enough practice, you'll come to have the list in your head, but that will take a while. Until then, have it available where you can read it, perhaps as a saved document on your smartphone or printed and taped to the door of the cupboard or fridge where your treats are kept.

Each item on your list offers a non-food reward (enjoyment, accomplishment, or both) in addition to buying you some time. They each redirect you toward activity that makes your life better rather than worse. The best case scenario is that the urge will pass altogether and you'll be happy with how you spent your time. The worst case scenario is that you'll white-knuckle your way through several alternatives from your list until the urge passes or you become legitimately hungry; I've strung them together for as much as several hours on a particularly tough day.

Or maybe the urge won't pass and you'll have to deal with it more directly (see below). Even then, at least you'll have gotten some beneficial things accomplished and will have spent that much additional time not eating, so you'll still be far better off.

What to Do When the Urge to Eat Just Won't Stop

Sometimes, no matter how mindful you are and how well you've set up your life so that you can be calm and controlled with food, it's still going to happen: that maddening, overwhelming, urgent desire to just *eat*, having nothing to do with physical hunger. There's no point in feeling like a failure when this happens, because it's very common. It still happens to me now and then.

You'll sometimes be able to identify what triggers it but sometimes, it will come for no apparent reason—as if a switch got flipped in your brain, causing you to become instantly obsessed with the need to eat. When this happens, it's important that you work through your bag of coping tricks very intentionally, doing whatever you can to restore some sanity or at least to minimize the damage. Amazingly, that switch in your brain will sometimes click off just as mysteriously as it clicked on—just like that, it's over, whatever it was. You'll be a much happier person if you manage to keep yourself at least somewhat together until the storm passes.

It's always a good idea at such times to recall past episodes like the one you're trying to avoid in the moment, re-experiencing the physical pain of the binge, the emotional heartache it created, and the days or weeks of negative ripple effects that followed. Then recall times like this when you somehow managed to dodge the bullet, whether it was by your own actions or because circumstances somehow shifted in your favor. Remember how grateful and relieved you felt afterward.

Do everything you can to trigger *emotional* memories that strengthen your resolve. Your emotional brain is the source of the current problem, but it also houses the power you need to make the best of the situation—you need to work with it as well as you can. Some days though, nothing is going to stop the need. You'll do your very best, and nothing will make a dent in it; it can feel like trying to stand up against a tidal wave.

Whatever happens, don't give up! If you've tried everything you know how to do and find that you're still hopelessly hung up on the idea of eating, keep your focus on maximizing safety and damage control. You are always in a position to minimize negative consequences, no matter what—always use that power in every way that you can.

There are two forms the need most often takes, and it's important to identify which of them you're dealing with so that you can choose the most effective strategy for managing it. The need might be for a specific food, or it might be the need to just eat, period.

If you think it's about a specific food, examine this carefully, because you might be mistaken. If it's the need to just eat *something* (which is often the case), you always want to be clear about that because the generic need to eat is easier to manage. When you've tried every way you can to outlast the urge, go ahead and satisfy it ... safely.

The way to do this is with emergency escape food. This is anything you can shovel down at will without doing too much damage because the food incorporates a lot of either water or air, thus giving it lots of volume yet comparatively few calories.

Vegetables fit the bill nicely in this regard, while offering a variety of tastes and textures to suit a range of cravings. You can keep yourself busy for a long time, get nicely full, and actually even get a bunch of nutrients that are beneficial anyway. If you feel the need to just mow through food for a while and almost anything will do, vegetables are an excellent choice.

My own go-to at such times is air-popped popcorn,[1] plain but for a sprinkling of popcorn salt (which falls off anyway since there is no oil to make it stick). It satisfies many different sensory needs because it's warm, it's got that hint of salt, it has a nice, carby crunch, and it keeps my hands and mouth busy for a long time.

My promise to myself has always been that when the tidal wave hits, I will munch without hesitation on as much of that popcorn as it takes, until I feel completely okay about stopping. Because popcorn with TV has always been built into my system anyway, I'll go ahead and watch TV too, because that seems to help.

Though I've always imagined having to go through as many as four large bowls of popcorn to get relief, the most it's ever taken has been two, and even that is rare. One will generally do it and then I am happily on my way, back to comfortably focusing on my life with no damage done.

If your overwhelming need has to do with a specific food, the first thing to consider is whether there is a less damaging alternative that is close enough in character to meet the need *effectively*. Think about which flavors and textures feel most important to you, and look for the safest way to get them. You'll probably need to do some experimenting in order to find substitutes that are truly good enough, but once you've identified them, you'll have your own go-to choices when the need hits.

Whether you identify a safer alternative or ultimately go for the target food itself, the next question will be: *What's the smallest amount of this that would satisfy my need?* This doesn't mean a token taste that would amount to little more than a tease. To be satisfied means to have had enough to meet the need without going any further than necessary; you're looking for the smallest amount you can eat that will result in your emotional brain eventually saying, *I'm okay now.*

An episode like this—even when actively managed—will be uncomfortable; the intensity and potential for loss of personal control can feel frightening. It will not be your finest hour. But if you keep working it the best you can, you can get through it with your dignity still largely intact and you'll be *very* glad for having done so. It's always worth making every effort that you can.

A client recently reminded me of a conversation we'd had in the past, comparing such episodes to being on a runaway train. Her words describe it best: "The train is bound to crash and burn at the end. You can jump off at any point. The further it goes, the more speed it picks up, and the harder it is to jump off. But it is never too late until the end."

Stay on Duty Whenever You're Around Food

Sometimes, you might feel like it would be a fine idea to take a break from being careful with food. Even if *you* don't feel that way, you'll sometimes encounter people who will tell you that you should.

"It's your birthday—you deserve to take a day off."

"Come on, live a little."

"This is part of the fun of the holidays."

"Hey, it doesn't hurt to loosen up sometimes."

These rationalizations will come to you at precisely the times when you are at the highest risk and can least afford to be off your game: situations that are or can easily become orange or red zones.

When you entertain such thoughts, it's your emotional brain talking. It can't see the danger. It can't see or care about the ugly consequences that will follow because those are too far in the future. It's being triggered and is beginning to react. You must reduce your risk as much as you can when you start to think this way, because it means you're one step from losing control.

If you don't act to keep yourself focused, you're probably going to end up hurting yourself with food and having regrets afterwards. Many people go off the rails for extended periods of time after an episode like this because it feels so demoralizing and hopeless—one bad thing tends to lead to another. You might manage it once without that happening, but you might not. It's a big risk to take.

Once again, consider driving. It's another activity we enjoy and which adds greatly to our quality of life, but which must be done with care because it always comes with a degree of risk. When does it ever make sense to take your hands off the wheel and your eyes off the road, no matter how much fun it might be to do something else instead?

Going off-duty for your birthday or any other special occasion is like taking your hands off the wheel and your eyes off the road when you're driving in terrible weather. It's an even worse idea than usual because the risk is so much greater. If you're driving, you have to keep paying attention no matter where you are. If you're tired of paying attention, you have to stop the car because the risk is simply too high to play it any other way.

Food in the modern world is risky for most of us now. If you're around food, you have to keep paying attention no matter where you are. If you're tired of paying attention, you have to get away from food because the risk is simply too high to play it any other way.

You might think this implies that you must suffer stoically, clinging to your carrot sticks and being a stick-in-the-mud at every party for the rest of your life, but that's not actually the case.

It means that when you're at a special event, you need to remember that you'll be encountering food in a higher-risk environment. You'll need to plan accordingly and keep focusing on doing your best, as discussed in Chapter 28. You'll probably end up eating a little differently from and a little more than usual due to the nature of the circumstances, but you can keep it from becoming a regrettable free-for-all.

Should you need more incentive for keeping your eye on the long-term prize at all times, consider this tidbit from the National Weight Control Registry, previously mentioned in Chapter 31. Those who manage two full years of consistency have a much higher rate of long-term stability with their behavior and therefore, their health. They just keep supporting the new neural pathways that take them where they most want to go, avoiding periodic "special occasion" blowouts that refresh the neural pathways associated with the dead-end results of the past.

Do Occasional System Checks

It's a good idea every now and then to step back and take an objective look at how you've been doing with food. Do you think you've been handling yourself mostly pretty well, or not really? Why? When are you at your strongest and most in control? When are you most likely to stumble and lose your focus? Has your life changed in any significant way—age, health, family structure, work situation, etc.—that means your system is in need of an update? What changes might fine-tune the system to make it more effective for you?

A system check is always a good idea in the wake of any lapse with food, even a small one. If you ended up making choices you didn't plan on and aren't happy about, you need to understand what happened so you can take action to keep it from happening again. Try to see what threw you off. If you got a do-over right now, what would you do differently in order to make it turn out better? How do you need to amend your approach going forward so that this particular lapse is much less likely to happen again?

I had to do a system check not so long ago myself. After a lovely holiday evening with dear friends, I realized I'd eaten too much spinach dip and cookies (no, not together). I would have had just as good a time *and* been more physically comfortable had I eaten less of each, so I was puzzling over why I'd done it.

I was chastened to realize that even after all these years, I'd made a classic rookie mistake: I'd simply stayed near the food too long. We were all having a grand time sitting around the dining room table, talking and laughing; of course, platters of goodies were on the table within arm's reach. At one point, someone even helpfully asked whether we should move to the living room where it would be more comfortable. "Oh no," I said, "we're doing great right here." Me. *I* said that.

The lesson *re*learned was that I need to get away from the food when I'm done with it so that I don't keep picking at it. I also realized that when I'm relaxing with people I love—even in the absence of food pressure—I'm at risk for relaxing a little too much around the food as well. My note to self for future times is to remember this and get myself the heck away from the food as soon as there's no longer any clear reason to be near it.

I felt better once I'd figured it out. I'm still learning, and this was another step in that process. I had a humbling reminder that those pesky neural superhighways of old are still operational if I wander onto one of them in a moment of inattention, but I also had a reminder of how easy it is to steer clear of them as long as I remember to do it.

If you make a mistake with food that causes you regret of any kind, don't waste time in self-recrimination—it simply doesn't help. If you could actually self-punish your way to better choices, it would have worked for you by now. In reality, self-recrimination is a painful, pointless process that is most likely to keep you out of control and doing more damage for a longer period of time. Rather than that, get to work immediately on figuring out what went wrong and why, and focus on how to fix it. That's what helps.

We all wobble sometimes. The gift of such times is that they show you where your system needs some work. Just put that information to good use, and your system will keep getting better and better. Like me, you might occasionally find that even the well-established parts of your system need some maintenance from time to time. No big deal. It's all part of the process.

Chapter 34
Pros and Cons of Some Familiar Strategies

As you adapt your food management tactics to the realities of today, you'll be dealing with your old ways of thinking and may initially want to keep using some of your old strategies, simply because they are what you know. Even now, you may feel the need to try them again, hoping that using them with your new perspective will yield better results.

They might have some utility for you going forward, or you might find that they pull you back into focusing on short-term manipulation of your weight rather than on long-term control of your eating. I can offer some observations about these strategies, gleaned from clinical conversations with the many people I have worked with who have tried them in the past. These are my personal impressions of the primary benefits and drawbacks of each, along with some suggested refinements or alternatives. I hope this assists you in making a more informed assessment of whether or how each of these strategies can fit into your system if you wish to consider them.

Accountability

I have heard many people express a belief that they need some form of accountability in order to stay on track. The chief practical benefit of accountability is that it adds some form of structure to your efforts, usually by way of milestone goals and specific timelines. As a result, it may enhance your ability to remain focused on the daily actions that will create the results you seek. If you enlist a friend as an assistant for accountability purposes, you'll have more contact and communication with that friend, which creates significant social and emotional benefits independent of your personal goals.

A downside to reliance on accountability is that it can be damaging to your self-concept. If you feel you must be held accountable in order to meet your goals, the implication is that you are untrustworthy and irresponsible, incapable of constructive action unless you are forced into it. In addition to being a bit of self-inflicted character assassination, it has great potential to inflame that whole *good-bad/should-shouldn't* problem with your emotional brain.

Another problem with systems of accountability is that they are usually time-limited, nowhere near long enough in duration to result in lasting behavioral and emotional change when it comes to food. The fledgling behavior usually gets dropped fairly soon after the system of accountability ends, and you're left with yet another failure experience.

I believe you can get the primary benefits of accountability with none of the pitfalls simply by using the goal pyramid described in Chapter 23. If you want to share your process with a friend, I suggest you do so in a manner that is based on support rather than enforcement.

Weigh-Ins

Since weigh-ins have been discussed in some detail previously, I'll add only a few additional comments here. It is important to remain aware of the status of your body and how it is responding to your eating and activity levels; many people value weigh-ins for this purpose. The scale gives them a reality check, helping them to detect changes in their weight before those changes have gotten too far out of hand. Many people would feel lost without the reference point provided for them by their bathroom scales.

On the other hand, weigh-ins keep you attuned to the reading on a device rather than focusing on and using feedback from your body. This concerns me because I believe that getting more attuned to your body—rather than less—is an important part of gaining more balance and control with food.

Another downside is that many people focus on the scale so much that they start doing unhealthy things like purposely starving and dehydrating themselves prior to a weigh-in; seeing the number go down (or rise less) becomes more of a priority than getting healthier and stronger. Many of these same people then go on to have a binge right after the weigh-in, because they "have a whole week" now before they have to worry about it again. That's just not a pathway to better health or personal peace, yet it's the path many take when they focus on the scale.

If you are among those for whom the scale is a mixed blessing, there is a highly reliable alternative method for staying attuned to your body: pants. Fitted pants with no elasticized panels or stretchy fabric, preferably with a high waist band. You need pants that stay the same size no matter what your body does so that as soon as your body changes at all, you'll notice it in how they fit.

If you don't have one already, get a pair of pants that meets these requirements and which *fits you comfortably as you are today*. There is so much stretchy fabric incorporated into today's clothing—even in jeans—that you may have to search some thrift shops or consignment stores to find what you're looking for. Pay close attention to exactly how the pants fit you right now.

Wear them for an entire day, noticing where they make comfortable contact. Notice any signs of tension in the fabric around your waist and hips when you have them on. Notice how they feel when you sit down, especially if you sit for longer than a few minutes. If you wear them with a belt, notice which hole in the belt you're using. Take actual notes on all of this if necessary, to assure that you have accurate baseline information.

Thereafter, try on the pants any time you want a quick spot-check on your weight, and commit to wearing them for at least one full day each week. With your detailed notes about every aspect of their fit and comfort at baseline, it will always be immediately apparent if something is changing, whether for the better or for the worse.

Pay special attention to how you *feel* about the prospect of wearing these pants for a full day at a time, especially for longer periods of sitting, because that will probably be your earliest sign that your body is changing. Even subtle losses of comfort will result in your liking the pants decidedly less; if you feel at all reluctant about wearing them, you're probably gaining weight. On the other hand, any weight loss will show up quickly as well, as you look forward to putting them on each time to see how much room you have.

This simple strategy will give you all the information you ever need. It's worth trying because most people react more rationally to changes in clothing fit than they do to every tenth-of-a-pound tick of the scale; as a result, this triggers fewer unhealthy emotional and behavioral reactions.

If you're not sure which strategy is best for you, consider an experiment where you try each of them. Use your scale for a month and then use the pants for a month. Don't be surprised if you feel nervous (maybe bordering on terrified) about going without the scale for even a short time; most people feel that way when they first try it. As you go through the experiment, take full notice of what you like and dislike about each strategy. You might settle on one or the other, or perhaps a combination strategy that takes advantage of the best of each.

Food Journals/Calorie Counting

Food journals can be beneficial in several ways. The most important one, in my opinion, is that documenting your actions can keep you more aware of what you're eating across the span of an entire day, as opposed to viewing each individual food choice in isolation from the rest. You can make better-informed choices when you see how each one fits into the big picture.

If you're paying enough attention to what you're doing to document every act of eating, then you're paying more attention to your eating in general, which is a good thing. You'll probably eat less food and eat more mindfully as a result. If you're using a journal app, you're probably getting lots of nutritional information on what you're eating as well, which can be a good reality check.

On the downside, many people find food journals annoying; if you feel emotional resistance to doing it, you probably won't stick with it for very long. It is common practice to skip entries that are deemed to be inconsequential, when the reality is that those little things add up in ways you'd never otherwise notice. Many people just cheat outright when they feel like breaking from their plan—they go ahead and eat what they want without recording it. Finally, if you keep your journal on an electronic device, you're spending yet more sedentary time with a screen and a keypad when you probably really need to be out engaging more with the physical world instead.

I would suggest as an alternative that you practice holding the memories of your day's eating in your head as you go along. You should, at any given moment, be able to recall what you've eaten and when. If you can't do this, it shows that you're eating too mindlessly to form usable memories. Since mindful eating is a vital skill in any event, this gives you an opportunity to practice it more purposefully. You can make a game of testing yourself a few times per day: *What have I eaten so far today and when did I eat it? How much did I have?*

You'll likely find that as you get better at keeping a mental record of what you've had so far, it will become easier to evaluate what and when to eat through the remainder of the day. This allows you to make each food decision in the larger context of the day, rather than as an isolated event. If you realize that the whole day has gone by with no vegetables, for example, you might decide to tilt dinner more heavily toward salad than you otherwise would have.

Since I've noticed that journaling food seems to trip people up more often than it helps them, I don't recommend it as a matter of course. There are occasions, however, when it can be useful on a limited basis. If, for example, you believe that your body is not responding even though you're eating well and moving adequately, a short-term, fully detailed journal of your choices can be quite illuminating.

Many of us have genuine perceptual distortions when it comes to evaluating how much we eat and how much we move. We tend to underestimate how much we're eating and overestimate how much we're moving, not because we're trying to fudge the numbers but because we genuinely believe it. Journaling is an effective way to get a more objective assessment.

I recall two people in particular who got quite an awakening as a result of journaling briefly when they felt stuck. Both were absolutely convinced that they had a clear view of what they were doing and were baffled by their lack of progress. Upon journaling, one elected to not share her findings with me, saying simply, "I see now where it was." The other, a woman extremely well-versed in nutritional information, was amazed to discover she had actually been ingesting *double* the number of calories each day that she'd guessed. Without a limited round of journaling, the mystery would have remained undiscovered, leaving both people at risk of feeling hopeless and giving up.

Sometimes, journaling to see why things aren't adding up actually shows perceptions that are reasonably accurate. If this is the case and what you're seeing just doesn't fit with what you're doing, it might be a good idea to get a medical check-up just to see what else might be going on. You never know.

Pre-Portioned Servings

I refer here to the prepared meals available through well-known commercial diet plans as well as the various 100-calorie snack packs now commonly available in your local grocery store. The obvious benefit of these is portion control, for which there is clearly a desperate need. Each one gives the consumer one less thing to think about, one less decision to make. This comes as a relief to many who are exhausted by how seemingly complex food has become. Another benefit is that these products provide a visual reference for reasonable portion size, which can be helpful.

A downside is that if you rely on others for portion control, you might remain dependent on external forces to provide the structure that you need with food. You need to be able to do this for yourself eventually, so if you do use pre-portioned servings, I hope you use them as a tool that enhances your learning rather than replacing it.

While pre-portioned servings may control for calorie count, there are no guarantees concerning nutritional value. A quick review of ingredient lists will show you that some of these products are highly processed; you know they're edible, but it's not as clear whether some of them are actually food in a sense that your body understands.

The 100-calorie snack packs might not be what you think, either. If you buy the 100-calorie pack of your favorite cookies, for example, look carefully at the ingredient lists and nutritional information of both the snack pack and the regular package of the same product. You may find that they are the same product in name only, and that the quality of the snack pack version is actually lower than that of its regularly packaged cousin.

Another noteworthy drawback to pre-portioned servings is that ultimately, there's nothing to keep you from eating several of them in one sitting if you choose. Many people have.

I recommend that you practice more active portioning on your own. You can do it more easily at meals with the help of smaller plates and bowls as mentioned previously. If you like the idea of snack packs, you can get them with less expense and higher quality if you package your own at home. A kitchen scale can be a useful tool if you choose to go this route, making it easier to size your portions appropriately and consistently over time.

Support Groups

There are many benefits to being part of a support group related to personal health goals. It's comforting to be among people of like mind, where your issues can be heard by others who can empathize accurately due to their own experience. Each individual has the opportunity to learn from the experiences and lessons of everyone else, potentially helping all to move forward with fewer unwanted detours. Knowing that you have a recurring group meeting to attend can help you to remain more mindful on a day-to-day basis the rest of the time.

On the other hand, all groups are not created equal; some function better than others at supporting the learning and progress of their members. The groups that I hear about tend to teach and promote a dieting mindset—often with an emphasis on weigh-ins—which is unsurprising since that's the way we've all been socialized. The problem is that the dieting mindset provokes resistance from the emotional brain and is therefore unhelpful for most of us. A group that is oriented toward dieting might keep you stuck in an approach to food that keeps ending up in the same unwanted place, over and over again.

Subtle balances must be maintained within a group to assure that it remains both healthy and helpful. Group members need to be supportive and empathetic, but not enabling; it doesn't help anyone if you all go down the drain together, everyone feeling wonderfully supported along the way. Group members also need to be very honest with each other, but without becoming confrontational or controlling. The best group will remain one of equals, avoiding our natural tendencies towards cliquishness, yet some leadership may be necessary in order to maintain focused, relevant discussions.

A highly functional group will make this all look easy, but never forget that it's a complex ballet of human interaction behind the scenes. A group that functions brilliantly this year may falter next year as the personality mix shifts with changes in membership. It's always a good idea to periodically reassess: *If I wasn't already in this group and was considering joining it for the first time today, what would I think of it? How am I now better as a result of the time that I've spent here? How does this group help me now? What do I need from this group going forward, and what do I need to do to maximize my chances of getting it?*

Two-Week Jump Starts

Many diet plans have a two-week jump start, a period during which you follow recommendations that are not typical of the remainder of the diet, and which usually claim to cleanse your system and/or give you a boost in rapid weight loss.

I haven't seen any benefit to these two-week jump starts other than that of emotional excitement. It's simply something new and different, which inspires hope. I've never known anyone whose eventual path to *long-term* success was kicked off by one of these, though in fairness, such a person would have no reason to contact me. On the other hand, I haven't encountered any of them in my personal life, either. In any event, some of these plans sound worrisome from a health standpoint and if you ever feel inclined to try one, I recommend that you consult with your doctor first.

This general approach seems to me to be about manipulating your body rather than partnering with it. I believe that way of thinking is part of the problem rather than the solution, so I can't recommend it. I suggest that instead, you keep your focus on quality food managed in ways that you can maintain for a lifetime. Combined with regular physical activity, this will allow your body's weight to normalize in a natural and sustainable way. It doesn't sound exciting, but it works.

Eliminating "the Whites": Refined Sugar and White Flour

The whites are prime ingredients in the foods that torment us the most: sodas, sweet treats, breads, crackers, many breakfast cereals, and many pastas. They are simple carbohydrates devoid of nutritional benefit, and every effect they have on your system is disruptive. They trigger addictive behavior from the emotional brain while creating extreme spikes in blood sugar and fueling the systemic inflammation that contributes to disease.

As a result, some people have attempted to eliminate the whites from their lives. In fact, total abstinence from both is considered a requirement for recovery by at least one well-known support organization, Compulsive Eaters Anonymous HOW (CEA-HOW).[1] This would appear to be a very straight-forward decision, given everything we now know.

I've spoken to a number of people who, at some point in the past, decided to do this on their own. Here is a reasonable aggregate of the stories told by every one of them: "Within a couple of weeks I felt *so* much better! I had more energy, I felt more clear, and I was in a much better mood. I couldn't believe how bad I'd felt before without realizing it. The change was amazing!"

And then at some point, each of these people gradually went back to the whites, generally returning to the painful patterns of their past.

I've spoken to a few people who made this effort in conjunction with joining CEA-HOW. All agreed that the program had a lot of merit, but none of them stayed because they felt that the requirements were too rigid. Each eventually dropped out of the program, returning fully—in the cases of those I've interviewed—to their old patterns of chronic overeating.

This puts us in a difficult position, because the only sensible thing to do is to step away from these substances completely, forever. It's the right thing from a medical standpoint. It's the right thing from an addiction standpoint. There appears to be no rationale for any other strategy.

Except that very few people seem able to do it long-term—most eventually go back. Having failed at their goal of abstinence, they give up completely (note the all-or-nothing pattern). They end up back where they started, but with one additional failure experience to add to their collection. I believe that fully abstinent people actually exist because I've heard of them from people I trust, but I personally can't recall ever meeting one in *any* context, whether personal or professional.

251

Abstinence from the whites appears to be impossible for the majority of us in our current environment; most emotional brains just won't stand for it while remaining exposed to opportunity so much of the time. The only way to escape fully from these foods would be to lock yourself up inside your own, safely stocked home, but that wouldn't make for much of a life.

Foods based on the whites are all around us in abundance, and they're not going away any time soon. Most of us have grown up with them and consider them a normal part of life. As much as we understand the problems associated with them, we still want them. We feel entitled to them.

Abstinence would be a simple solution—just don't touch any of the stuff. The decision-making doesn't get any cleaner than that and it would bring nothing but benefits to your health. If you can manage it without resistance from your emotional brain, it's the way to go.

If your emotional brain can't handle abstinence, however, there's still hope. It might be possible for you to include some of these foods in a limited, carefully planned way that allows you to embrace the healthier choices you need to be making the majority of the time.

It's a delicate balance which can easily become too precarious if you're not working at it *very* carefully. You need to retain just enough of these treats to keep your emotional brain happy, but you must avoid being triggered into uncontrolled eating and you must assure that you don't consume enough of them to generate any negative health effects.

Finding this balance is tricky; maintaining it takes ongoing attention and effort. If you're willing to make that effort and understand that you can never get complacent about it, you might find that it actually helps you to stay on track for life. My own story is instructive in this regard.

I had my awakening with food in 2001, and immediately set about creating a new system for myself. My new patterns with food had to keep me both happy and healthy, while protecting me from the risk of lapsing back into compulsive eating again. It was obvious to me from the start that if I tried to eliminate everything involving the whites, my system would quickly collapse. I just knew it. I could *feel* it.

I didn't understand the brain science of all of this at the time. I just knew it would be foolish to construct a system with an obvious auto-destruct feature. I realized that if I *planned* for one such snack every day, I could feel okay about focusing on nutritious eating the rest of the time. I understand now that my emotional brain can accept waiting for the treat as long as it knows when the treat is coming.

I quickly found that the treat needed to be placed at the very end of each day. If I tried having it early (e.g., someone brought goodies to work), it always felt like the emotional party was over while there was still an awful lot of day left. Even though I tried to tell myself that the treat for the day was now done, I'd feel an overwhelming desire for the usual treat later on anyway.

If I simply wait until the evening, however, my emotional brain is perfectly happy with nutritious food all day long, and then it's also happy with the treat later. It can still get triggered by unexpected circumstances midday but if I can make it through that, I'm always very happy to have escaped unscathed, and then to thoroughly enjoy my snack later without feeling out of control.

When I first started this in 2001, I quietly hoped that someday, my interest in the snacks would diminish. I wasn't going to force it in any way, but knowing the nutritional realities of this stuff, I thought a life without it would be a nice end result. As of 2016, it has not yet happened. I feel much less urgency about these foods now, but if I even consider outlawing them altogether, I can still feel the stirrings of an internal revolt. After many years of a better relationship with food than I would ever have thought possible, I'm okay with letting it ride. It's working quite well.

That said, I'll be the first to tell you that I have to work at managing myself with these foods now just as I did at the very beginning, whereas all other foods have gotten pretty easy at this point. If you're willing to do the work, and understand that you will *always* have to do the work when it comes to such foods, *and* you think it's worth all that effort, there can be a place for some of them in your life. If that's what it takes to keep your emotional brain on board with your goals, it might be what helps you to stay on track for good.

You are likely to find that some foods are so triggering for you that it's simply easier to walk away; some tasty treats just aren't worth the work that is required to enjoy them safely. Your best bet for finding middle ground that works—treats that keep your emotional brain satisfied without exposing it to undue risk—is to eliminate those foods that predictably pitch you into the orange or red zone. Identify treats that you can enjoy in the yellow zone provided you plan for circumstances in which it is reasonably easy to maintain control, and with the understanding that you must always be as mindful as possible when you have them.

You'll quickly learn through experience which foods strengthen your system and which ones destabilize it. You must be brutally honest with yourself about what you can handle and what you can't, retaining *only* those foods that you can manage and which you find to be worth the effort. Otherwise, it's only a matter of time until it all falls apart again. You've already been through enough of that.

When it comes to the whites, you have three options, each with a noteworthy drawback:

- You can change nothing, which means you're likely to remain out of control with food for the rest of your life.

- You can choose abstinence, which is usually sustainable only if you can do it without resistance. You'll probably only be able to embrace abstinence if you're feeling so destroyed by your compulsion for these foods, that you know in your heart you can only be truly happy if you escape them completely. The problem is that some resistance is the norm and if you feel any of it, you are likely to abandon abstinence at some point.

- You can practice controlled use of triggering foods, which requires ongoing mindfulness and care. Do it well and managed use of those foods can actually be part of a happy life. Get complacent and your emotional brain will quickly spiral out of control. It's admittedly a razor's edge to walk.

My own path did not involve the conscious assessment of these options because I didn't comprehend all of this enough to understand the choices at the time. I instinctively knew that certain foods would always take me somewhere I could no longer stand to go, but I never swore them off. I just stopped thinking about them because I could finally see them for the dead ends that they'd always been.

As for the treat foods I've kept, I've concentrated on figuring out *how* to have them so that I can have the enjoyment with minimal risk. That has meant having them in small portions, and only at times and in places where I feel confident that I can maintain control. I simply don't have them any other way except occasionally in social situations, and then only with great care.

There are several key themes to my experience which are worth considering as you chart your own course. I've put my focus on what *to* do rather than fussing much over what not to do. I spend my time looking forward to and planning for the foods that give me the life that I want, which simply leaves less time and energy available to think about the foods that would throw me off track.

I never swore off the whites, yet their presence in my life is negligible; they simply got pushed aside in favor of foods that do a lot more for me. It's been more about adding new options than about taking anything away. The more I fill my life with things that make it better, the less room there is for anything else. It's a nice, resistance-free way to go.

Chapter 35
Beyond Overeating

You may wonder, after everything you've now read here, what it all actually amounts to in real life. If you make the kinds of changes you see described in these pages, will you be glad you did? Will life still be enjoyable enough?

If you are able to shake the dieting mindset you've probably had for years—a considerable challenge in itself—and use this new information to refine your approach, you are likely to experience a number of pleasant surprises.

Nice Surprises About Food

The biggest surprise may be that you are likely to enjoy food more than you have in a long time—maybe ever. The most obvious benefit is that the less you overeat, the less you experience guilt, shame, regret, physical misery, and long-term health problems. If all you achieved was to reduce painful results like these, your quality of life would dramatically improve, but that's just the beginning.

You will enjoy your food more because you'll be paying more attention to it as you eat. You'll notice the flavors and textures in much greater detail, rather than having them sail through your mouth virtually unnoticed as is the case when you're eating mindlessly. Because you'll notice the experience with more appreciation, you'll be able to feel genuinely satisfied with smaller quantities than you've required in the past.

I, for example, used to plow rapidly and urgently through half a large, loaded pizza (six big slices) until I couldn't possibly stuff down another bite. Once I began to see and use food differently, I realized that when shoveling down half a pizza, there was little of it that I had actually noticed. I'd unconsciously found it necessary to keep eating more so that I could notice enough of it to feel like I'd really had the experience. I have since found that when I'm paying attention, eating slowly, savoring every bite, it only takes two slices to feel like I've had the full pizza experience. I get more actual enjoyment (because I'm paying attention) out of two slices than I ever got out of six, plus I don't feel horrible when I'm done. This is unbelievably better, I can assure you, and my experience is typical. This is a reliable outcome if you stick with the approach that makes it possible. Lapsing back into mindlessness with food is the only thing that takes this away.

The example above sets you up for the next nice surprise. You can be quite successful and happy in this new way of life with food even as you continue to enjoy some foods that frankly do not top any nutritionist's list of recommendations. Realistically, of course, it won't work to have them at nearly the frequency or quantity to which you've been accustomed—you've done that experiment and it has ended badly, just as it always will.

There's a little room for food that's purely for fun, however, and you'll get the most mileage out of it by paying full attention when you eat it. The only exceptions to this are those foods that are so triggering to you that it's impossible for you to enjoy them in a managed way that creates only good outcomes. The reward of fun food deteriorates quickly the moment anything bad begins to come of it, so you need to avoid any foods that might trigger you into going too far.

Speaking of triggering foods, another nice surprise is that you are likely to lose your interest in some of them. Most of my clients eventually come to see some of their past favorites as "gross"—the word they most frequently use—when they begin to see those foods as blobs of sugar, fat, salt, and mystery substances somehow congealed into a form that's convenient to eat.

It's a lovely thing when a food that has called your name for your whole life suddenly goes silent, forever. That won't happen with all such foods, unfortunately, but it will probably happen with enough of them to make your life considerably easier going forward.

Whether you are surprised by the foods you discover you can eat with control or by the ones that no longer torment you, they are all good surprises.

The Gift of Learning Your Limits

A more successful life with food means acknowledging and respecting your personal limits. These are not limits that restrict what you can have, which is an artifact of the dieting mindset. These are the limits within which you know you can maintain control and free will, enjoying both your food and your dignity. When we stay within our limits, we can relax and enjoy ourselves, creating only good memories along the way.

If we exceed our limits, we act in ways we later regret, whether physically, emotionally, or both. Regret of any kind is one of the clearest signs that a limit has been exceeded. In the moment of regret, we would give anything to go back in time and be able to stop just *before* we hit the limit, but we can never undo it once it's happened. The secret is to respect your limits in the first place; using them effectively means maximizing your good times, not detracting from them.

You'll find that the concept of limits also applies to various practices; some practices will work for you and some won't. For example, you might be able to keep some tempting foods in your home without suffering a loss of personal control, but not others. You'll probably identify a number of foods that you can enjoy with control at certain times or in certain circumstances, but which become risky for you otherwise. Some foods might be okay for you while watching TV, but if you're like most people, it won't be many. Some foods might be safe for you when you're alone, while some probably won't.

Perhaps you can maintain your mindfulness more in some social situations than in others. Or maybe you'll find that you can hold it together at any type of social gathering as long as you don't attend a lot of them, or if you limit how much time you spend when you go. Most people find that it's much harder to observe their limits with food when they're drinking alcoholic beverages. Many foods that are fine for you under normal circumstances will become unsafe for you when you're stressed.

It may seem complicated when you consider the various limits we have and how they fluctuate based on internal and external circumstances. The reality though, is that you'll figure yours out fairly easily once you start really paying attention.

It's simple—each time you feel regret, you've just discovered the location of another limit. You'll know that this time was an example of "too far" or "didn't work," so you can make an educated guess for doing better next time. Eventually, you'll have your limits fairly well mapped out and won't have to give them much ongoing thought. As you develop stronger habits for sticking with what works, you'll have more and more energy available for simply enjoying and appreciating your life.

It Keeps Getting Better

The longer you keep at this, the better you'll feel. Since you'll be approaching your life and eating patterns in a way that takes the best care of all parts of you, including your emotional brain, you won't be quietly seeking escape. It isn't that you'll never wobble; you almost certainly will, but it's likely to happen less often and less intensely over the years.

You'll enjoy clearer thinking, greater personal peace and integrity, a stronger, healthier body, and a much happier relationship with food. You'll probably lose your tolerance for feeling less than your physical and emotional best, which will strengthen your motivation even more.

You'll refine your practices over time, gradually honing an approach that works smoothly, effectively and with maximum satisfaction for you. You won't get it all figured out right away and you'll probably find that you need to fine-tune it periodically as your circumstances change, just as you do with other aspects of your life, but you'll get there. Someday, you may find that it no longer feels like a different thing that you're doing, but that it has simply become part of who you are and how you go through life.

Your personal process may go fairly smoothly, or not so much. It may gel quickly or seem to take forever to come together. Your weight may adjust to what you're hoping for or it may not. Regardless, you're likely to find that being on the road to getting better—even with potholes and detours—still feels better than being out of control.

I attended a seminar on nutrition some years ago, during which one of the speakers—while dispensing the usual guidelines for dieting—asserted, "Weight control is a lifelong project." While I did manage to contain myself, what I wanted to do was jump up and yell, "No! *Life* is a lifelong project!"

Life is about living. It's about growing and learning, loving and surviving grief, taking chances and learning to move forward through challenges, and about discovering how to be who you really are. It's about laughing and crying, singing and dancing. It's about playing, creating, sharing, and contributing. And at some point, it's about leaving, hopefully with a sense of having spent the time reasonably well. To look past all of that in favor of a narrow focus on weight is tragically to miss the point of making the most of our one, magnificent shot at this life. Perhaps the best thing about this new way of living with food is that you get to focus far more of your energy on *living*.

May you live very well, indeed.

The Challenge of Evenings

If you're busy during the day and find it especially hard to maintain control with food in the evening, you're not alone. There are several reasons that evenings are difficult for most people who operate on a fairly conventional schedule.

First, you may be emotionally spent by the time evening comes. Having dealt with various challenges and obligations since morning, you're now hoping to downshift and relax, at least a little. You have less focus now than you've had all day, which makes you vulnerable.

Next, you probably spent most of the day on a schedule, knowing where you had to be, when you had to be there, and what you were supposed to be doing at the time. You've gotten through all of that and have finally made it to the evening; your time is now more your own. This is the least structure you've had all day which, while welcome, adds further to your vulnerability.

You're tired and you want to relax. You want comfort and reward, and you've earned it. Plus, you're probably going to spend some time camped in front of the TV, which seems to trigger the munchies in most people. Uh oh.

But that's not all.

Evenings are when the demons come out to play. If you're lonely, depressed, grieving, worried, anxious, or otherwise struggling, the evening is when you're likely to feel it the most because there's so much less to keep you busy and distracted. Unless you've found a more constructive way to take care of yourself when you feel unsettled, you're likely to seek solace in food, munching your way through the evening until you can hide even more effectively in sleep.

Maybe now you can see why evenings are so hard. You're vulnerable in several different ways all at the same time. Fortunately, there are several strategies for making them somewhat easier in terms of control with food. The strategies are simple ones, each with the potential to help to at least some degree.

- It helps to have something to do with your hands while you're watching TV, especially if your activity requires you to keep your hands clean. Common choices include needlework or other crafting, puzzles, doodling, coloring, or minor household tasks like folding laundry.

  If you find any of these activities to be appealing, but too distracting to be pursued while watching TV, that makes them ideal choices for ways to spend non-TV time. Anything that really captures your attention will reduce your yearning for food by keeping your mind otherwise occupied.

- Some people find it beneficial to simply stay away from the kitchen after a certain hour. Some take it a step further and avoid rooms adjoining the kitchen as well, for an extra margin of safety.

- For many of us, the psychological boundaries of the evening are defined by two specific events: when dinner ends and when it's time to go to bed. It is the span of time between those two points that triggers so many of us into whiling away the time by grazing.

  Consider simply shortening that span. If you eat dinner a little later and/or go to bed (or at least retire to the bedroom, perhaps for reading) a little earlier, you effectively shorten the length of time during which you are most vulnerable. Shortening it by as little as 30 minutes is enough to make a difference that you'll appreciate.

- If you eat during the evening, consider snacking only on your emergency escape foods during that time. You'll get the soothing effect of munching behavior without the high-calorie burden of more conventional snack food.

- You might find it enjoyable to sip on a cup of caffeine-free tea in the evening, as long as that doesn't result in extra bathroom trips later on that disrupt your sleep. Tea has warmth and flavor, while providing a lot of the same, soothing hand-mouth behavior that you get from eating. It might well be enough to keep you content, for at least part of the time.

- If you have some flexibility in how you schedule your time, try to shift as many activities and commitments as possible into the evening hours. This will keep more of your free time oriented toward the daylight hours when you naturally have more focus and control.

Strategies like these will not completely solve the problem of wanting to eat all night long, but they'll make evenings easier for you, which is probably the best we can hope for. I don't know of anyone who ever struggled with evenings to start with (there are actually a few who don't) who ever got completely free of it.

I haven't. Evenings are the only hard part of my day at this point. The rest of it generally flows quite nicely, but I've got to be mindful and cautious every night, even now.

It's okay though. Evenings spent being careful are making me a lot happier than evenings spent out of control ever did, and I suspect you'll find the same.

Appendix B
Considerations for Restaurant Buffets

Restaurant buffets have been quite popular for some time now, and many restaurants have them. Buffets allow you all the self-serve convenience of eating at home, but with a much wider variety of options and the ability to walk away from it all at the end without leaving a pile of dishes in the sink.

Buffets may not have been designed specifically to prompt overeating, but they might as well have been. The book *Mindless Eating*, by Dr. Brian Wansink of Cornell University, is a priceless resource in understanding why this is so.

The problems with buffets begin with where we find them: in restaurants. As mentioned previously, restaurants themselves are highly triggering places in any event. There are sights and smells of food all around, occurring in an environment that *has* been designed specifically for the purpose of encouraging you to eat.

Buffets confront us with a large quantity of food. This is a setup for overeating because we tend to eat more when there are greater amounts of food available.[1] They also offer us a wide variety of choices, another setup for overeating because we are triggered to eat more overall when we have more options.[2]

These two elements—quantity and variety—combine to force us into *many* food-related decisions in a short period of time, all while in a very triggering environment. The opportunity for costly mistakes could hardly be greater.

When we serve ourselves from a buffet, we are surrounded by others who are going through the line and loading up their plates. This stimulates us to unconsciously do the same, since we tend to mimic the behavior of those around us.

Finally, we all like a good deal. The price of most buffets is fairly economical compared to ordering from the menu, but it's astoundingly economical if you eat as much as you possibly can. Buffets create a financial incentive to overeat: the more you eat, the more food you get

264

for the money you've spent. It can feel wasteful to eat less than physically possible.

For all of these reasons, buffets are generally best avoided if you wish to remain in control of your eating. While the meal you order from a menu will probably still be oversized, at least there will be some limit to the food made immediately available to you.

If you decide to tackle a buffet anyway, you might be able to reduce your risk somewhat by making your decisions beforehand. The goal would be to make your decisions with your cortex ahead of time, rather than doing it with your emotional brain while all that tasty food is right in front of you. The risk remains high even then though, because your emotional brain is likely to take over once you get to the buffet anyway.

If you're going to eat at a buffet, here's a thought strategy that might help. Think of the buffet not as a chance to get the most food for your money, but as a chance instead to get the *perfect meal* for your money. The perfect meal will include samples of everything you really want, in serving sizes that—when added together—leave you satisfied but not stuffed.

This only works if you are able to eat slowly despite the triggering environment, and if you are able to stop at some point despite the fact that you could physically eat more if you decided to. Remember that you won't really know how full you are until 20 minutes later; given the unique hazards of buffets, you probably need to make a point of quitting extra early just to be on the safe side.

If you continue eating after your body has had enough, you start creating the bad results that detract from the reward value of the meal. It might feel like you're getting more food for your money, but you're actually paying a high price for it in unnecessary emotional and physical discomfort.

Appendix C
Safer Enjoyment of Special Occasion Meals

Here is the sequence of events experienced by many who overeat (and some who usually don't) when it comes to anticipating a special occasion meal. They look forward to it with great anticipation. They eat very little early in the day so as to have lots of room available for all that great food later on. They dress in loose or stretchy clothing, knowing that anything else will become painfully tight before the end of the evening. They reassure themselves that special events like this are no time for being careful about food because that would take all the fun out of it.

By the time the event begins, they've been fantasizing about the food for hours and are very, very hungry due to having eaten too little during the day. They begin eating with great urgency, loving the food but actually noticing relatively little of it because they are eating so rapidly. They stop eating only when they have to because they actually can't fit in another bite. They feel bloated and uncomfortable, but will probably still go for dessert or a later snack despite remaining overly full from the main meal. They have trouble getting to sleep that night because they are so physically uncomfortable from overeating.

They awake the next morning with little hunger for breakfast because they're still full from the night before. They look back on the event with mixed feelings—it was fun and the food was so good, and yet it would be nice to not have overdone it so much. It would be nice to feel better the next day.

If you've read the book up to this point, you can now easily see the many ways in which our typical approach to such events sets us up for self-abuse with food. There is another way and if you do it, you can enjoy yourself, enjoy the food, and sleep well that night. You can wake up the next morning comfortable and refreshed, with no regrets and no need to do any damage control. You can then get on with your life without the interruption of unwanted consequences.

These results can be yours if you're willing to try some new ways of approaching special occasion meals. It's important to remember that the goal is not to deprive yourself of enjoyment, but to save yourself from regret and discomfort. In order to do that, you need to be able to maintain enough control with food to keep acting in your own best interests. To do *that*, you need to remain aware of what you're doing and why, with specific care about which foods and how much of them end up in front of you (since you're likely to eat them once they're there).

In Preparation for the Event
It starts at the beginning of the day, and it starts with taking care of yourself exactly the same way you do every other day. This means eating a good breakfast and just as hearty a lunch as usual, to keep yourself properly fueled and to keep your body functioning in its normal rhythms. As long as you don't overeat at these earlier meals, you will be plenty hungry enough to enjoy yourself by the time the event begins.

It can be helpful to remind yourself that when it comes right down to it, this dinner is just another meal. You had dinner yesterday and you'll have dinner tomorrow—this happens to be what you're having for dinner today. It doesn't have to be a reason for frantic excitement—it's just a nice meal. It's easier to maintain control when you remain calm.

This, of all days, is a good day to exercise. Not in a desperate attempt to get ahead of all those extra calories you're afraid you're going to eat, but to keep yourself thinking clearly and feeling in touch with the body you'll want to protect once things get started.

Dress in clothing that makes you feel good about how you look. Such clothing will probably be at least somewhat fitted, which means that you'll feel it if you overeat. Knowing that your clothing can get tight won't prevent you from overeating, but it's one small, additional limit which might help you to remain more mindful.

Consider providing your own escape food, perhaps a generous vegetable tray with a flavorful, low-fat dip. This will give you an out if, at some point, the triggering nature of the event leaves you overwhelmed with the urge to start shoveling food; if you need to shovel, do it with veggies. Who knows? There might be someone else there who appreciates having a safe option as well.

As you look forward to the event, purposely keep your thoughts on the social aspects of it rather than on the food. Who will be there?

What conversations can you look forward to having? What conversations can you make a point of starting? Who might you make a point of getting to know a little better? This will help to reduce your focus on the food, which will help with managing the urges. Better yet though, it gives you something much more important and meaningful to think about instead.

During the Event
There tends to be a lot of free-choice food at gatherings like this, so consider strategies that naturally help you to eat with more control:

- Put everything you eat on a plate, no matter how small the item is. Even if it's just a cashew, put it on a plate before you eat it. This will keep you mindful of what you're doing and will help you to slow down. It will also help you to assess the importance of each food item. If it's not worth the trouble of putting it on a plate, is it worth eating at all?

- Use the smallest serving dishes that are available, because larger dishes automatically trigger more eating. Smaller dishes make it easier for you to remain content with less food (Chapter 32).

- Take *small* samples of everything you think you'll really enjoy, remembering that all those small samples will add up to a lot of food if you're not careful. Most people underestimate how much they're eating and the likelihood is that at an event like this, you'll still overeat to some degree despite your best efforts. By purposely aiming low in the quantities that you take, you can reduce the degree to which that happens.

  It's best to try to avoid overeating in the first place because once you've done it, you're stuck with it. On the other hand, if you actually manage to eat too little (unlikely, but theoretically possible), you can always go back and get more.

- Remember that the flavor of the food has less impact as you continue to eat. The way to get the maximum flavor hit from everything is to keep the portions small.

- Once you've made it through your first round, remember that you've probably already consumed a noteworthy amount of food. It's good to pause a bit before going back for any seconds, to give yourself a chance to see how your body feels.

If you do go back for more, consider doing so only for the one or two items that you love the most.

Try taking a little less than you think you really want and then give yourself some time to see how you feel after you've finished it, because you'll probably end up satisfactorily full after all. If not, you can always go back and get more. You have plenty of time; there's no need to rush.

- Consider saving your very favorite food for last, if you think this might motivate you to save room for it by not loading up on everything else first.

- Take control of your portions. Don't hesitate to cut a small piece or take a small sample of something that has been pre-portioned for you. It does no harm to take just part of it, and there's a good chance someone else will be happy to have the small piece you left behind.

- Consider eating with your "other" hand for part of the time, or at least with your most challenging foods. The point of this is not to annoy you into eating less (though it may have that effect). The point is that you are not accustomed to eating with that hand, so you will be very aware of every little thing that you're doing. Awareness helps you to choose more mindfully and eat more slowly.

- Focus on taking small bites, savoring them fully. Think about nibbling your way through the food rather than attacking it, remembering that the more slowly you eat, the more enjoyment you get out of each bite.

- Try to avoid eating when you are highly distracted, such as while in the midst of an animated conversation. Simply stop eating until things slow down, and then go back to it with appreciative attention when the time is right. Why bother eating delicious food when you're too distracted to notice it?

- Beware of heavy, fat-laden dips. They are highly triggering, with little nutritional value but many, many calories. If you choose to indulge, think about using such dips as an accent for the food rather than using the food as a shovel for the dip.

- Socialize away from the food as much as possible. Sit or stand somewhere else whenever you reasonably have the opportunity to do so. You'll find it far easier to manage yourself if the food is in the next room rather than within arm's reach. Keep your focus on the people around you, and it will be easier to think less about the food.

- Stay physically near and purposefully aware of anyone present who seems to be eating with moderation. Because we are influenced by the behavior of those around us, you'll find it easier to slow down if you pace yourself on someone else who is eating with control.

- Be mindful of how alcohol affects you and consider drinking a little less at an event like this rather than more, as is the usual practice. Aside from the obvious problem of the empty calories in alcohol, nobody gets *smarter* around food when they drink.

  You might find it helpful to bring along flavored sparkling water. This is a festive drink option which sidesteps both the empty calorie and impulse control problems associated with alcoholic beverages. You can enjoy it as is, or use it to reduce the alcohol and calorie content of your drinks by making wine or juice spritzers.

- It's helpful to drink water part of the time, regardless. It keeps your mouth and hands busy when you might otherwise casually grab some food, and helps you to pace yourself. Remember to use the trick of taking a big gulp of plain water to rinse off your taste buds when you're trying to resist the urge to go back for more food.

Strategies like these allow you to enjoy yourself, enjoy the food, remain physically comfortable, and fit into the same clothes the day after that you fit into the day before. It's all good. You have to work it purposefully to get things to turn out this way but if you do, you can enjoy special occasions more than ever before.

Appendix D
Hosting Special Occasion Meals

In Appendix C, the emphasis was on actions you can take to maximize your enjoyment of food during special occasions, minimizing your risk of overeating to the point of discomfort and regret. Some of these occasions, of course, might take place in your own home. The great advantage to this is that when you are the host, you set the tone for the event. You are in control of the variables that determine whether the food experience—for yourself as well as your guests—is a relaxing and safe one, or whether it is fraught with triggers that challenge self-control.

Here's what people often say after a special dinner at the home of loved ones: "I had a wonderful time, but I ate way too much and felt really stuffed all night. I wish I hadn't done that." Here's what they *could* say: "I had a wonderful time. I usually end up eating way too much at these things, but this one was different. I really enjoyed everything, and I actually felt great at the end of the evening. What a nice change."

How do you want *your* guests to speak of their time in your home after the gathering is over?

Changing the Focus
As you prepare for your gathering and invite your guests, you begin to set expectations for the event based on how you describe it. The common practice is to make it all about the food, with enthusiastic descriptions of all the wonderful dishes and treats that will be shared. It's implicitly understood that getting together is meaningful, but all that really gets discussed or described is the food.

If you prime yourself and your guests to focus on the food, everyone will focus on the food. In your case, that means you will set up an atmosphere that is highly triggering. What it means for your guests is that they will arrive already overly focused on eating. The outcome for everyone is predetermined before the event ever starts.

Alternatively, you could shift the focus of attention. What if there was an implicit understanding that a meal would be part of the event, but that what you most discussed and anticipated was how you would spend the time together? When you set the tone *this* way, food is a supporting player rather than the star attraction; you and your guests can gear up for the event by thinking more about each other and less about the food.

If you're like most people, you've been making your gatherings all about the food for so long that it might be hard to imagine doing them any other way. As mentioned in Chapter 30, even small groups of people tend to do very well at brainstorming for new ideas, so you might get a kick out of doing this with your loved ones. If you have to tackle it on your own, however, you might find yourself getting stuck. In case you need some ideas to get you started, here are some that have been offered up by my clients and seminar participants:

- General conversation and catching up, of course!
- Share family videos.
- Share photos and tell stories.
- Make another activity—movie, play, concert, visiting a local attraction—the central focus of your gathering, enjoying a simple meal together afterward.
- Walk together before or after the meal.
- Backyard activities like bocce, volleyball, horseshoes, croquet, Frisbee, badminton, hopscotch, bean bag toss, or hula hoops.
- Hike together or just enjoy the sights at a local park, sharing something simple for dinner afterward.
- Make crafts together for personal use, for donation to others, or for getting a head start on holiday gifts.
- Puzzles—big ones to be done as a group project.
- Indoor games (many creative ideas are available online).
- Write letters to US military personnel who are away from home.
- Make gift baskets or boxes for donation (shelters, nursing facilities) or to send to US military personnel.

- Volunteer together (soup kitchen, food bank, local shelters/missions, litter pickup, etc.) and trade stories about the experience afterward over a casual meal.

Having developed some other ways to focus everyone's energy and attention, the food part will naturally be less prominent—not *gone*, just not the primary focus. This will pave the way for your next challenge as a host bravely trying new strategies, which is to gauge the success of your event not on how much everyone eats or how much they like the food, but on how much they enjoy themselves overall. This has probably always been in the back of your mind anyway, hiding behind your conscientious concern about providing an excellent meal for your guests. Just move it to the front of your mind instead, confident that your guests will still eat just fine even if you all think about the food a little less than you used to.

More Relaxing Ways to Feed Your Guests
The default for many hosts is to provide lots of food from beginning to end: snacks, appetizers, elaborate meals, and dessert. On top of all of that, many guests bring additional food in order to contribute.

Between the host who over-prepares in order to avoid running out of anything and the guests who bring even more, the end result can be an overwhelming amount and variety of food which predictably stimulates us to eat more than we want or intend.[1] It's kind of fun in a chaotic way while it's going on, but then everyone lies around feeling sluggish and uncomfortable for the rest of the evening, with many continuing to feel out of sorts into the following day.

You as a host can set things up to turn out differently. If you are willing to experiment with some new approaches in presenting food, you are likely to find that you and your guests actually enjoy yourselves *more* overall. A good goal would be to enable your guests to enjoy your food without being influenced in any way to go too far. They still *can* overeat, of course, but you can create an environment in which they do so entirely of their own accord rather than in response to triggers set up by you.

Most gatherings feature food presented in an opt-out fashion. It's right in the front of the guests at all times so that if they don't want it, they have to make a point of ignoring it at close range over an extended period of time. While the ability to opt out does technically exist, the emotional brain is likely to be so triggered by all the easily available food that opting out is difficult, at best. Few people seem able to manage it.

On the other hand, an opt-in environment will leave your guests in much greater control of their actions. With an opt-in environment, your guests know where the food is and are free to help themselves as they wish, but it's not always right in front of them. They will find it a few extra steps or a room away, rather than having it constantly at their fingertips.

Your guests' emotional brains (and your own) will certainly still react to the general proximity of special food but if you have to make even a slight extra effort to see or get to it, that allows your cortex some room to work. As a result, everyone is more likely to have an enjoyable evening that ends very well, rather than getting caught up in a high-speed food fest that ends in discomfort and regret.

If you're game for trying this new approach, here are some tips to help you along, addressing each element of the meal.

Food Brought by Guests

Many of my clients, working as they are to be calmer and more in control around food, find that the easiest option for them is to take charge of all of the food for the gatherings that they host. This way, they are in control of both the quality and quantity of food available to everyone, managing the level of triggering associated with each. It's more work this way but you might find that it makes for an emotionally calmer time for you, allowing much easier self-control with food.

When you ask your guests to bring nothing but their charming selves, some will ignore that request and bring food anyway, believing that it would be inconsiderate to do otherwise. Unfortunately, the food they bring is often exactly what you're trying to avoid, for your own purposes if not that of your other guests. My clients who have faced this situation have incorporated the food into the event at such times in order to be kind, followed by insisting that the guest take home whatever remains of the food that they brought. If the guest refuses, the leftovers are discarded.

An alternative is to let guests know what you could use, being specific about both the type and size of the dish; for example, "a vegetable dish of about ten servings." You can coordinate everyone's efforts so that when it all comes together, it is a meal of reasonable proportions for the number of people in attendance. Some guests will happily go along with this, while others will still bring either too much of what you requested or something else entirely.

You can only make your best effort and then manage the actual results as well as possible. The weight of our traditions in this area is substantial—it's going to take a sustained effort over a *long* time to effect real change.

Snacks and Appetizers

Many people consider it good hosting to have snacks readily available for guests, staging bowls of munchies at every location where anyone might congregate or sit. This is meant to be an act of generosity but as noted earlier, it is an opt-out situation which few emotional brains can manage.

Some people genuinely prefer to wait for the meal, but it's really hard to *not* absent-mindedly munch while chatting ahead of time if the goodies are always immediately at hand. It is certainly *possible* to resist the temptation, but it is difficult and distracting. Few people actually succeed at it.

If you wish to provide snacks for those who truly want them, the opt-in strategy is to have the main supply of munchies somewhere slightly out of the way but easy to get to, with individual bowls available so that guests can serve themselves as they wish. This way, those who opt in will do so because they *want* to, rather than being unable to opt out because their emotional brains are too heavily triggered by having snacks set up right next to them.

I recommend keeping appetizers minimal, if you serve them at all. Many people serve appetizers that are practically a meal in themselves, essentially forcing their guests to overeat by the time dinner is added to the mix. If you must have appetizers, try having enough for everyone to have a liberal taste, but not much more. Don't worry, there's a whole meal coming—everyone will be fine. In fact, they'll be *more* fine if they're not full before dinner even begins.

Veggie trays do nicely for anyone who wants something before dinner. They generally aren't triggering, so those who partake of them are likely to do so out of choice rather than compulsion. This is the aim of providing an opt-in environment: creating a space in which people can eat calmly because they want to, rather than eating chaotically because they can't stop themselves.

Dinner

Here too, the goal is to create a calm and relaxing experience for everyone (including yourself), in which it is possible to eat with at least some degree of self-control. Happily, everything you do toward this end will also reduce the work associated with hosting, so you'll get benefits above and beyond calmer enjoyment of your food.

- <u>Reduce the total amount of each item that you prepare</u>. The vicious cycle of hosting is to make excessive quantities of everything in order to ensure that there is enough, and then to pressure everyone to eat too much in order to keep the extra food from going to waste.

  If you prepare everything based on reasonable meal portions and the desired amount of leftovers, it's likely to work out just fine. If one or two things happen to run out, there's more of everything else. It will be okay.

  This benefits your guests because they won't feel the pressure of an excessive amount of food, and it benefits you because it lightens your workload in the kitchen. Everybody wins.

- <u>Reduce the number of different dishes that you prepare</u>, remembering that the more options we have, the more we tend to eat. Make multiple vegetable dishes, if anything, avoiding heavy sauces. Beware of overloading with simple carbohydrates as we do for the typical holiday meal that includes some form of potatoes, bread-based stuffing, *and* dinner rolls. The more such items you present, the more important it is to do so in small quantities that don't invite overeating.

- <u>Downsize your dinnerware</u>. This will help everyone with natural portion control as they fill their smaller plates. Your guests can go back for more servings at any time, so smaller dishes do nothing to restrict eating—they just make it easier to slow down and choose a bit more thoughtfully. Heavy-duty, decorative paper plates are good for this because their wide rims naturally leave a smaller usable area for food.

- <u>Portion carefully when you're doing the serving</u>. Some platters or baking dishes are too hot or too heavy to move around the table, or the table may simply be too crowded to allow for their being passed around. At such times, it may be necessary for you to serve your guests individually. When you do, ask each guest what they would like, and how much. Then, do your best to honor their requests as accurately as possible, assuring that you don't give them more than they asked for. If they want more, they'll let you know.

- Don't prompt any individual to take larger or additional servings, trusting that your guests will take or ask for more if they want it. A no-pressure way to assure that everyone has gotten enough is to ask general questions like, "Does anybody need anything?" or to remind the group that everyone is welcome to help themselves to anything else that they'd like.

- Model a relaxed pace throughout the event. Special occasions tend to result in near-frenzied eating by the group, to no one's real benefit. Since people are influenced by the behavior of those around them, you can help the whole group to go slower and enjoy the food more mindfully by doing so yourself. If you have difficulty with this, scan the room to see who is eating most slowly, and then pace yourself on that person. Even if only a couple of people eat at a calmer pace, it will be easier for others to unconsciously follow suit.

  When everyone slows down, three great things happen. Your guests get more enjoyment from their food, they're able to more fully appreciate your time and effort in preparing it, and they're more likely to end the evening feeling comfortable rather than bloated. Again, everybody wins.

- Clear the table at the end of the meal. It is common for groups to chat around the remnants of dinner for some time after everyone has finished eating, which results in a lot of mindless picking at leftovers. Nobody really cares about doing this because they're already full from dinner. They just do it because the presence of the food continues to trigger them. It makes everyone's life easier if the food just disappears after they've had enough.

Dessert

It makes little sense to offer dessert right after dinner, when no one is hungry. In any event, eating when you're already full is the perfect definition of overeating, and you're trying to help your guests steer clear of that. If it feels too strange to simply delay dessert until later—perhaps because this flies in the face of time-honored tradition—the best of both worlds is to make dessert available for anyone who does want it right away, while planning on another opportunity later for those who prefer to wait.

Pre-portioning dessert for your guests is a good idea only if you make the portions very small. This facilitates easy portion control for everyone because they can take multiple small portions if they wish, or mix and match different samples if there is more than one dessert on hand. Otherwise, it's best to let everyone serve themselves, assuring that small dessert dishes are available for that purpose.

It's good to be careful about the total number of desserts available, by the way, as desserts often multiply beyond reasonable proportion to the number of guests in attendance at a gathering. This matters because abundance and variety will trigger your guests into overeating as they attempt to avoid missing out on all those special opportunities. It is far easier for everyone if the amount of dessert available is kept at a manageable level in the first place.

Don't Worry, It'll be Okay

You can expect to feel uncomfortable about trying some of these new ideas simply because they are different. This is how most of us reflexively react to change, especially when that change challenges well-established patterns and especially when those patterns carry sentimental or symbolic meaning.

Your discomfort might show up as concern that you're being a negligent or stingy host, but a quick reality check will reassure you that this is not the case. The fact is that you will still be providing your guests with plenty of food and caring attention.

What you *will* be providing less of is environmental pressure to overeat. That's all, and that's a good thing, because nobody likes pressure. The result is an experience for everyone that is calmer, more relaxing, more comfortable, and more enjoyable. Many of your guests will continue to struggle with their own food issues (whether you know it or not), but at least you can provide a setting that supports them rather than exploiting their vulnerability.

Changes like those suggested here create a *better* food experience, not a lesser one. If you doubt that, try it and see. If you don't like how the experiment turns out, there's nothing to prevent you from returning to your old practices if that's what you prefer.

If you do like how it turns out, it will help if you make some notes for yourself about the experience: what you did, how it worked, how it felt, and what you thought about it immediately afterward. This is important because the next time you decide to entertain guests, you'll tend to revert back to your previous habits (old neural pathways, of course) unless you give yourself a clear reminder of exactly why you liked the new ways when you tried them.

Your old habits are likely to be so strong that you'll need to go through this process of reminding yourself each time you have guests, possibly for the rest of your life. It will be worth it though, because you'll end up enjoying yourself more every time, and so will they.

Appendix E
Considerations and Strategies for Travel

Travel can be a welcome break from all the usual home routines, allowing you a change in scenery that supports a nice mental reset. However, travel is also likely to disrupt most of the patterns that help you to stay safe with food under normal conditions.

When you're dealing with different people, surroundings, and circumstances than you're used to, you're likely to experience both the loss of some valuable anchor points and the introduction of new, more challenging triggers.

Many people respond to this by abandoning their efforts for the duration of their trip, with the intention of getting back on track once they get home. This allows for a lot of damage in the interim though, and such people often arrive home feeling bloated and sluggish. For many, however, that's not where it ends. Having thrown caution to the wind while away, they can't find it again once they get back. The trip is often just the beginning of weeks or even months of unstructured, mindless eating, often at a level that wipes out any progress toward health goals that had previously been made.

For these reasons, it is advisable to maintain your efforts as best you can when traveling, realizing that you're going to have to improvise along the way. You might not manage the level of success you enjoy at home, but you'll still come home in far better shape—both emotionally and physically—than if you make no effort at all. With that goal in mind, here are some general tips to get you started.

Focus on Keeping Your Focus

From the moment you begin making your plans, make your trip about *the trip*, rather than about the food. Direct your attention and anticipation very purposefully toward the special opportunities that you'll have: the people you don't normally get to see, the places you'll get to visit, the activities you'll get to enjoy, and the simple pleasure of a break in your usual routine.

Once your trip is underway, make it a point to really *be* there, noticing everything and committing the experience to memory. Doing this will help you to enjoy yourself more fully while also keeping the food triggers from hitting you quite so hard. Don't worry if you find it necessary to purposefully refocus your attention in this manner many times, perhaps quite frequently. You probably will. The important thing is that it will improve your experience of the trip every time.

Ideally, you'll eat in ways that enhance your experience of the trip, without going too far and creating regret. Just keep doing your best, knowing that it will be challenging. Don't ever give up. Travel is difficult because it's a deviation from your normal patterns, but it's also of limited duration—you won't have to maintain the additional level of effort for very long. No matter how badly you might struggle at times, there are always things you can do to minimize the damage, and Future You will be grateful that you did.

When you eat, it will help if you intentionally prioritize your body's nutritional needs. This will bias you towards the whole foods that have what you need and which are less likely to tilt you into overeating. As always—and even more so on a trip—exercise great caution around foods that are highly triggering. Momentary temptations quickly come and go, but regret and shame drag on for a very long time.

More than ever, you'll benefit from slowing down your eating so that you can really notice your experience of the food. This will be harder than usual due to the different circumstances in which you find yourself, but the benefit you get from doing it will be that much greater as a result. This will give you a more full experience of any special foods that are not usually available to you, as well as making it easier for you stay in control.

You can protect your personal peace and integrity only if you purposely choose options that lift you up rather than pulling you down. When faced with challenging decisions about what and how to eat, consider questions like these:

- *Is this likely to make me stronger and happier? If not, what is it likely to do instead?*

- *How many times have I done something like this and then been glad that I did? How many times have I done something like this and then wished that I hadn't?*

- *What would I think of this choice if I knew someone else was struggling with their eating as I do, and I saw them making it? Would I think they were celebrating life in a way they'd remember fondly, or would I think they were losing control in a way they'd probably regret later?*

Finally, pay special attention to how you end up feeling each day after you've managed to keep your focus with food to at least some degree. You'll know you're making the right calls and missing nothing of value if you end up feeling calmer and more at peace—maybe even relieved—rather than frustrated, stressed, or disappointed. This is an outcome you can create as long as you hang in there and keep working the situation as actively and intentionally as you can.

Tilt the Odds in Your Favor
Your primary strategies will be different depending on whether you are staying with loved ones or venturing out on your own for a business trip or vacation.

Staying with People You Know

When staying in the homes of others, communication and gentle assertiveness are essential. Your hosts can't possibly know your needs if you don't articulate them, so look for opportunities to help them help you.

If your hosts are like most people, they'll focus on making sure they feed you well while you're with them. Do all you can to remain in control of your own portion sizes, and be prepared to politely decline food offers that are not in your best interest, even if you have to do so repeatedly. You don't need to go into any long, personal explanations—just keep kindly saying, "No, thank you," while reassuring your hosts that you're getting plenty to eat and are enjoying their company.

Much of this kind of visiting ends up being focused on talking and eating, so don't hesitate to offer up ideas for sharing the time that are about activities rather than food. Most people are quite open to such ideas once they are offered—it just isn't the first thing many people think about on their own any more. Because there is deeper bonding value to shared activities than there is to shared food anyway, your ideas might mean that you all enjoy each other's company even more than you otherwise would have.

At the very least, you can try to gently influence everyone to settle in and chat in areas of the home that are less food-oriented than the kitchen table, for example.

When You're Away on Your Own

An important principal for eating away from home is to minimize the number of times that you have to make food decisions spontaneously. As at home, this requires planning. Unlike home, you have considerably less control over the variables in play, so you just have to do the best you can with what's available.

If the circumstances of your trip permit, it's always advantageous to take along some of your own food. Breakfasts are the first challenge and can easily become rather heavy affairs, especially if you go to a buffet. I personally just plan for breakfast in my room, having brought along my usual cereal along with some instant milk that I prepare for it each morning. This means I can keep having the breakfast I'm accustomed to (so, no new triggers there), and I'm not even dependent on having a fridge in the room for milk. A plan like this might not be of interest to you, but I like it because it means every day gets off to a healthy, calm start. It gives me a nice boost of confidence for the rest of the day as I venture forth into the unknown.

It's also good to bring along your own snacks, chosen based on your ability to stay in control when you have them. Many fruits and vegetables can hold up well for a few days; good selections include anything that is kept unrefrigerated in your grocery store's produce section. Dry cereal is good for crunchy munching in the evening if you need it, and protein bars are a reassuring hedge against an outbreak of real hunger once you've retired to your room for the night. When you know you don't have to fear going hungry later on, you don't have to load up on dinner just to be on the safe side, nor do you have to grab some high-calorie goodie from a vending machine, convenience store, or even room service simply because you lack other options.

Being away from home necessarily means eating out. Since you have no choice but to do it and you'll have to do it many times over the course of your trip, it will turn out better for you if you figure out how to handle it before you go. This means doing some research ahead of time to find out which restaurants are available at your destination, and checking out nutritional information on their websites (if possible, depending on where you're going) so you know which choices will work for you. To the extent that you can make food decisions like these before you go, you will have fewer such decisions to make once you're there where conditions are so much less favorable for it.

In an odd twist, domestic travel creates a unique situation in which national chain restaurants can be a helpful option. Though much of their fare can be problematic, they generally have a few options that can work as long as you've dug into the nutritional information enough to find them. Because chain restaurants provide the same dining experience wherever you go, knowing what to expect will spare you from being triggered by novelty in unfamiliar surroundings. Offerings might differ between locales even within the same chain so it's good to confirm, if you can, that your preferred selections are available at your destination. When in doubt, it's good to have some backup options in mind just in case.

If you're feeling disappointed at the idea of eating the same old things while traveling that you're already accustomed to, remember that food is not the point of your trip. If you keep the food part of your travel more predictable (less triggering), keeping your emotional focus on everything else about your time away, you're less likely to end up so out of control in your eating that you can't get back on track once you return home. The sweet spot you seek is to eat in ways that add to your good times without creating problems you'll have to live with once the trip is over.

You can certainly make exceptions for special local fare if your destination warrants it, but just be aware that your risk is significantly higher in unfamiliar places and with unfamiliar foods. Any time you wander from the patterns that you know, you'll have to work harder at managing yourself in order to enjoy your meals without lapsing into choices that cause you later regret. When you want to try a special food, aim for the smallest serving size that will allow you to feel like you've really had the experience; anything beyond that will be potentially harmful excess.

Wherever you eat and whatever you choose, beware of ordering large meals when you have no meaningful way to take advantage of leftovers. This might happen either because you don't have a fridge in your room or because your plans just aren't conducive to meals of leftovers. If you have no way to make use of the extra food, you're likely to feel compelled to try to finish your oversized meal in order to "keep it from going to waste."

It's far better to do all you can to assure that you start with a reasonably sized meal in the first place, which might mean ordering a senior's portion, half portion, an entrée to split with someone else, or an appetizer to serve as your meal. If you manage to end up with too little food, you can always order more. Wouldn't *that* be an interesting change of pace?

Happy travels.

Appendix F
A Word About Bulimia

My apologies to anyone who has gone all the way through this book, hoping and waiting for help that is specific to bulimia nervosa (commonly known as bulimia), only to find that it is not addressed here. If you're not clear about what bulimia is or whether it is an issue for you, it is a pattern of overeating which is accompanied by compensatory behaviors performed for the purpose of preventing weight gain.

These behaviors include self-induced vomiting; misuse of laxatives, diuretics, or enemas; fasting; strict dieting; or excessive exercise.[1] The DSM-5, published by the American Psychiatric Association, defines bulimia as "mild" if compensatory behaviors are performed an average of one to three times per week, with increasing degrees of severity assigned to increasing levels of frequency.

My clinical experience has been with those who overeat and whose practice of the above behaviors is, at most, limited and infrequent. Those are the people whose needs I understand the most, and with whom I feel capable of providing competent help. My writing is specific to them because they are the people I really know.

Many overeaters have occasionally dabbled in compensatory behaviors without adopting them in any consistent way. If this is as far as you've ever gone, I urge you to avoid going any further. These behaviors have medical risks, including that of becoming an additional addiction. It's just best to not tempt fate.

If you think that bulimia has become a problem for you, everything in this book will be useful as regards the overeating part of your patterns, but I recommend that you seek additional help for getting the compensatory behaviors under control.

If you don't know how to locate these services in your area, you can contact the National Eating Disorders Association (NEDA) at their website: http://www.nationaleatingdisorders.org. You'll find lots of educational information there, along with a list of healthcare providers in your area.

I urge you to reach out for help if you think you might need it. You don't need to struggle alone with this for even one more day.

Join the Conversation

You are invited to join the Facebook group page for readers of *Why We Overeat and How to Stop*. It has been established to give you a forum in which to explore the material further if you wish.

This is an online community where you can get support, ask questions, and discuss anything you need to in order to move forward more effectively. The group is open to anyone on Facebook, but posts are visible only to members of the group. All members are authenticated by the moderation staff prior to admission.

The page will be moderated only as needed to ensure that it remains a safe, informative, and inviting place for discussion, free of marketing and other off-topic posting that detracts from the focus of the group.

You can find the group at the URL below. If you have any questions or have difficulty finding us, you can contact me through my personal Facebook page or my website, www.elizabethbabcock.com.

Come visit at:
www.facebook.com/groups/1706869689594710/

Acknowledgments

Writing this book has been a remarkable experience. I had to ask quite a few people for information and assistance along the way, and since I wanted the material to be the best it could be, I asked all the best people I know (go big or go home). Such people tend to be very busy, so I hoped I would be lucky enough to find a few who would say yes. As it turns out, almost *all* of them did.

All were very generous with their time despite the fact that most of them really didn't have it to spare—they just made it work, somehow. Some offered personal or professional insights, while others offered technical assistance. All made my job a lot easier and the book a lot better.

Jennifer Britton, on staff at Drexel University, is part of the team managing Drexel's neighborhood initiatives. She has no time available for the demanding job of editing, but stepped right up and did it anyway. She assisted with everything from the earliest brainstorming sessions to the detailed refinement of every last page, offering excellent suggestions, observations, and critiques that resulted in considerable improvements to the text. She's been a great friend for what is now a surprising number of years; adding this project to our list of shared adventures has been the gift of a lifetime.

Dr. Evgeniy (Gino) Shchelchkov, a board certified neurologist, graciously agreed to review my earliest draft. His validation of my approach gave me the confidence to forge ahead over the many months of writing that followed. That he also took a personal interest in the book and reviewed it once it was finished was an unexpected and much appreciated bonus.

Diana Heaton, Laura Amend-Babcock, Linda S. Flemmer, RN, Sheila Bowtle, EMA, and Sally Ann Fleming all generously agreed to be beta readers, each giving me an early reader's-eye view of the material which helped me to work out some rough spots and improve clarity. Janet Russell assisted with the final proofing; she and Ms. Heaton served double duty as the official grammarians of the project, which was a tremendous help. If you see anything in the text that is written improperly now, you can be sure that it's because I kept noodling around with it after they'd worked their magic. Some of us, you see, just can't be left alone to write without adult supervision.

Debra Bates, RN, is the Director of Health Ministries at Christ United Methodist Church in Bethel Park, PA. She has actively supported my community education efforts for some time now, was a tireless cheerleader throughout the project, and continues to work to increase local awareness of this book's message.

Many other healthcare professionals generously agreed to post reviews of this material. You'll find excerpts of their thoughts at the beginning of the book, and their reviews are available in full on my website. They each took many hours of precious personal time to read this book as a favor to me; thanks to their efforts, potential readers can get some idea of why this information is worth a look when so many other options are available. Special additional thanks go to Katherine Stephens-Bogard, MS, RDN/LD, CDE, RYT who went above and beyond the call of duty as a reviewer to offer valuable suggestions which improved the material further.

Many clients have allowed me into their worlds over the years, each adding—in their own ways—to the knowledge base that made this work possible. Therapy group members in particular have contributed a great deal; you'll see their input in the helpful lists that appear in Part Four.

Last but certainly not least, there is Jim, the epitome of partnership and an unfailing source of support in all things, who waited patiently as I focused enormous amounts of time and energy on this book for 18 months of our lives. I owe him more than I can say.

I am beyond fortunate to have so many caring and talented people willing to step up and make both my world and this book a lot better than would otherwise be possible. Thank you, all.

Notes

Preface

1. Gregory Boothroyd and Lori Boothroyd, *Going Home*, (Delton, MI: Greenwood Associates, 2005). This is the most updated version of the book, while the one I originally learned from was in print at the time as *Goin' Home*.

Chapter 1—The Deep Desire to be Normal

1. Cynthia Ogden, Margaret Carroll, Brian Kit, and Katherine Flegal, "Prevalence of Childhood and Adult Obesity in the United States, 2011-2012," *Journal of the American Medical Association* 311:8 (2014): 806—814. Available at http://jama.jamanetwork.com/article.aspx?articleid=1832542 (accessed March 25, 2015).

Chapter 2—So Much Eating

1. As chef Anthony Bourdain memorably stated in an interview for TIME magazine (August 17, 2015: 60), "We used to get together with our friends to see a movie, after which we'd go have dinner to talk about the movie. Now we just go straight to dinner and talk about the dinner. And we take pictures of our food while we're doing it."
2. More detailed information on this point is available in numerous texts on childhood development. It has also been conveniently summarized on the CDC website at http://www.cdc.gov/ncbddd/actearly/milestones/index.html (accessed April 25, 2015).
3. CDC, "Do Increased Portion Sizes Affect How Much We Eat?" Research to Practice Series, No. 2 May 2006, http://www.cdc.gov/nccdphp/dnpa/nutrition/pdf/portion_size_re search.pdf (accessed March 21, 2015).

Chapter 2 (continued)

4. Brian Wansink, *Mindless Eating: Why We Eat More Than We Think* (New York: Bantam Books, 2006): 59—60.
5. Ibid., 71—75.
6. USDA, "Food-Away-from-Home," October 29, 2014, http://www.ers.usda.gov/topics/food-choices-health/food-consumption-demand/food-away-from-home.aspx (accessed March 21, 2015). Research data referenced in this report is available at http://www.ers.usda.gov/data-products/food-expenditures.aspx.
7. For additional information, see David Kessler, *The End of Overeating: Taking Control of the Insatiable American Appetite* (New York: Rodale Inc., 2010). This book is essential reading for anyone trying to create a manageable relationship with food.

Chapter 3—So Little Food

1. While the spirit of this statement is true, it must be noted that there are still far too many people in the US who, for various reasons, do not yet have reliable access to quality food. The issue of hunger and food insecurity in some segments of our population is beyond the scope of this book, but remains a very real concern.
2. This was captured in great detail in "The Flavorists: Tweaking Tastes and Creating Cravings," a *60 Minutes* (CBS News) segment originally aired on November 27th, 2011. The video can be seen at http://www.cbsnews.com/videos/the-flavorists-tweaking-tastes-and-creating-cravings. The script of the video can be viewed at http://www.cbsnews.com/news/the-flavorists-tweaking-tastes-and-creating-cravings-27-11-2011/. It is a remarkable piece of work that should be studied carefully by anyone who buys food prepared outside the home. Admittedly, that includes essentially everyone in the developed world.
3. David Kessler does a great job of exploring this in detail in *The End of Overeating: Taking Control of the Insatiable American Appetite* (New York: Rodale Inc., 2010).
4. More information about the Guiding Stars program is available at http://www.hannaford.com/content.jsp?pageName=GuidingStars&leftNavArea=HealthLeftNav.
5. Bill Jeffrey, "Health Check Program," *Canadian Medical Association Journal* 178:9 (April 22, 2008): 1187—1188. Available at http://www.cmaj.ca/content/178/9/1187.3.full (accessed April 21, 2015).

Chapter 3 (continued)

6. Federation of American Societies for Experimental Biology (FASEB),"Highly processed foods dominate U. S. grocery purchases," *ScienceDaily* (March 29, 2015). Available at www.sciencedaily.com/releases/2015/03/150329141017.htm (accessed April 2, 2015).

7. Ken Ashwell, *The Brain Book* (Buffalo, NY: Firefly Books, 2012): 188. The author notes evidence suggesting that use of language dates back at least 40,000 years, and that language is how we transmit knowledge between people and across time. This provides a useful approximation for when humanity's herd knowledge of food began to develop.

8. Far more detailed exploration of this issue can be found in Michael Pollan's *In Defense of Food* (New York: Penguin Books, 2009).

Chapter 4—Still Life

1. Ian Wyatt and Daniel Hecker, "Occupational Changes During the 20th Century," *Monthly Labor Review* (March 2006). Available at http://www.bls.gov/opub/mlr/2006/03/art3full.pdf (accessed April 21, 2015).

2. Mayo Clinic, "7 benefits of regular exercise," February 5, 2014, http://www.mayoclinic.org/healthy-living/fitness/in-depth/exercise/art-20048389 (accessed March 28, 2015).

3. CDC, "Physical Activity and Health," February 16, 2011, http://www.cdc.gov/physicalactivity/everyone/health/index.html?s_cid=cs_284 (accessed March 28, 2015).

4. Holly Wagner, "Use It Or Lose It Rings True When It Comes To Exercise," *Ohio State Research News* (April 2004). Available at http://researchnews.osu.edu/archive/userlose.htm (accessed April 21, 2015).

5. Brooke Salzman, "Gait and Balance Disorders in Older Adults," *American Family Physician* (2010). Available at http://www.aafp.org/afp/2010/0701/p61.html (accessed March 28, 2015).

6. Garry Egger, "In Search of a Germ Theory Equivalent for Chronic Disease," *Preventing Chronic Disease,* 9 (2012): 110301. Available at http://www.cdc.gov/pcd/issues/2012/11_0301.htm (accessed April 21, 2015).

Chapter 4 (continued)

7. Eric Ahlskog, Yonas Geda, Neill Graff-Radford, and Ronald Petersen, "Physical Exercise as a Preventive or Disease-Modifying Treatment of Dementia and Brain Aging," *Mayo Clinic Proceedings*, 86:9 (2011): 876–884. Available at http://www.ncbi.nlm.nih.gov/pmc/articles/PMC3258000/ (accessed March 28, 2015).
8. Aviroop Biswas, Paul Oh, Guy Faulkner, Ravi Bajaj, Michael Silver, Marc Mitchell, and David A. Alter, "Sedentary Time and Its Association With Risk for Disease Incidence, Mortality, and Hospitalization in Adults: A Systematic Review and Meta-analysis," *Annals of Internal Medicine,* 162:2 (2015): 123–132. Available at http://annals.org/article.aspx?articleid=2091327 (accessed April 26, 2015).
9. _____, "The Benefits of Physical Activity," *Harvard School of Public Health Nutrition Source,* (2010). Available at http://www.hsph.harvard.edu/nutritionsource/staying-active-full-story (accessed April 26, 2015).
10. Neville Owen, Genevieve Healy, Charles Matthews, and David Dunstan, "Too Much Sitting: The Population-Health Science of a Sedentary Behavior," *Exercise and Sport Sciences Reviews* 38:3 (July 2010): 105–113. Available at http://www.ncbi.nlm.nih.gov/pmc/articles/PMC3404815/ (accessed April 26, 2015).
11. S.J. Lees and F.W. Booth, "Sedentary Death Syndrome," *Canadian Journal of Applied Physiology*, 29:4 (August 2004): 447-460.

Chapter 5—Living Longer, Aging Faster

1. Elizabeth Arias, "United States Life Tables, 2010," *National Vital Statistics Reports* 63:7 (2014). Available at http://www.cdc.gov/nchs/data/nvsr/nvsr63/nvsr63_07.pdf (accessed April 22, 2015).
2. Robert Fogel and Dora Costa, "A Theory of Technophysio Evolution, With Some Implications for Forecasting Population, Health Care Costs, and Pension Costs," *Demography* 43:1 (1997): 49—66. *Demography* is published by the Population Association of America.
3. CDC, "Prevalence of Overweight, Obesity and Extreme Obesity Among Adults: United States, 1960-62 Through 2011-2012," September 19, 2014,

Chapter 5 (continued)

http://www.cdc.gov/nchs/data/hestat/obesity_adult_11_12/obesity_adult_11_12.htm (accessed April 23, 2015).

4. S. Olshansky, D. Passaro, R. Hershow, J. Layden, B. Carnes, J. Brody, L. Hayflick, R. Butler, D. Allison, and D. Ludwig, "A Potential Decline in Life Expectancy in the United States in the 21st Century," *New England Journal of Medicine* 352:11 (2005): 1138—1145. Available at http://www.nejm.org/doi/full/10.1056/NEJMsr043743 (accessed April 22, 2015).

5. Paola Scommegna, "Aging U.S. Baby Boomers Face More Disability," March 2013. Published online by the Population Reference Bureau, available at http://www.prb.org/Publications/Articles/2013/us-baby-boomers.aspx (accessed April 22, 2015).

6. Ibid.

7. CDC, "Childhood Obesity Facts," December 11, 2014, http://www.cdc.gov/healthyyouth/obesity/facts.htm (accessed April 22, 2015).

8. Mayo Clinic, "Childhood Obesity," April 10, 2015, http://www.mayoclinic.org/diseases-conditions/childhood-obesity/basics/complications/con-20027428 (accessed April 22, 2015).

Chapter 6—The Obvious Question

1. National Institutes of Health, "Sodium in diet," May 13, 2014, http://www.nlm.nih.gov/medlineplus/ency/article/002415.htm, (accessed March 25, 2015).

2. David Kessler, *The End of Overeating: Taking Control of the Insatiable American Appetite* (New York: Rodale Inc., 2010): 3—64.

Chapter 7—It's All About Your Brain

1. The information in this chapter is widely available in many sources covering structure and function of the brain. Ken Ashwell's *The Brain Book* (Buffalo, NY: Firefly Books, 2012) was selected as the core reference here because it is a fairly user-friendly book for the general public, including nicely detailed illustrations which provide a clearer sense of how the parts of the brain are arranged. Page numbers for various specifics are provided for anyone who may wish to explore in more detail.

Chapter 7 (continued)

2. Ibid., 17, 40.

3. Ibid., 34–35. If you desire more technical detail on this part of the brain, the main terms to research are limbic system, amygdala, hippocampus, hypothalamus, and basal ganglia.

4. Ibid., 223, 244.

5. Ibid., 187.

6. Ibid., 20, 215.

7. The brain is incredibly complicated, with many areas of minute specialization working in tight coordination to allow us to live the complex lives we enjoy. The parts most relevant to the understanding of eating issues lend themselves to fairly easy generalization, but please know there is so very much more.

Chapter 9—Six Important Things to Know About Your Emotional Brain

1. Jamie Oliver, a well-known chef and food educator, once showed young children how chicken nuggets are really made. The children were disgusted by the raw ingredients (admittedly with a bit of egging on by Mr. Oliver), yet readily said they would still eat the nuggets if given the opportunity. This is a classic case of pre-existing love for the food overruling new information to the contrary. The video can be seen here:
   https://www.youtube.com/watch?v=pPnKxWvPM6o   (accessed July 29, 2015).

2. George Koob's *How the Brain Forms New Habits: Why Willpower is Not Enough* is an educational program for healthcare professionals which is published and sold by the Institute for Brain Potential (IBP) in Los Banos, CA. If you don't mind a more technical discussion of the brain, you may find it a useful addition to the material in this chapter. The CDs or DVDs for the course (recently retitled as *Calming an Overactive Brain: How the Brain Forms New Habits*) can be purchased directly from IBP.

3. Ken Ashwell, *The Brain Book* (Buffalo, NY: Firefly Books, 2012): 232.

Chapter 11—The Key to Living Well in Today's World

1. S.M. McClure, D.I. Laibson, G. Loewenstein, and J.D.Cohen, "Separate Neural Systems Value Immediate and Delayed Monetary Rewards," *Science* 5695:306 (October 15, 2004): 503–507. This study looks at the interplay of the two brain systems in decision-

Chapter 11 (continued)
making; an interesting discussion of the study can be viewed at http://news.harvard.edu/gazette/2004/10.21/07-brainbattle.html (accessed January 26, 2016).

Chapter 12—The Fallacy of Normal
1. Alcohol is not considered here since it is not a core beverage used throughout the day for the primary purpose of hydrating.
2. Nick Hall, *Preventing and Managing Chronic Inflammation, Special Focus: Nutritional Interventions*, (Los Banos, CA: Institute for Brain Potential, 2015). This is a continuing education course for professionals, available on CDs or DVDs purchased directly from the Institute for Brain Potential.
3. Ibid.
4. Ibid.
5. Mayo Clinic, "Diseases and Conditions—Constipation—Risk Factors," August 31, 2013, http://www.mayoclinic.org/diseases-conditions/constipation/basics/risk-factors/con-20032773 (accessed December 30, 2015).
6. Cleveland Clinic, "Diseases and Conditions—Constipation," 2012, https://my.clevelandclinic.org/health/diseases_conditions/hic_con stipation (accessed December 30, 2015).

Chapter 14—Fear of Getting Nutrition Wrong
1. Most people adapt quite easily to whole-grain breads and cereals, while some are initially put off by the firmer texture and more robust flavor of whole-grain pasta. After having the pasta a few times, most find it to be quite satisfying. The refined pasta products they once cherished then come to seem mushy and flavorless by comparison.

Chapter 15—Critical Misperceptions
1. OECD, *Health at a Glance 2013: OECD Indicators*, (Paris: OECD Publishing, 2013): 42, 58. This report can be accessed at http://dx.doi.org/10.1787/health_glance-2013-en (accessed October 11, 2015).
2. The noteworthy exception to this is any food you find so intensely triggering that it is simply not possible to have any of it without losing control of your ability to choose. Such foods trigger the emotional brain into a takeover, overriding the cortex's reasoning abilities and resulting in personal loss of control. Most people can

Chapter 15 (continued)

identify some specific foods that they know they will probably never be able to manage with true enjoyment and dignity. Some foods just aren't worth the trouble it would be to try find a way to make them work, if it's even possible. However, that still leaves many, many choices to savor and enjoy.

3. Many thanks to JM for sharing this priceless bit.

Chapter 16—Misuse of the Brain in Decision-Making

1. While 95% is the failure rate perhaps most frequently cited, it's hard to find a credible, recent source to verify it. In the case of my clients at least, it appears to be true.

Chapter 18—The Body of Your Dreams vs. the Body in Your Mirror

1. C. Ochner, A. Tsai, R.Kushner, and T. Wadden, "Treating obesity seriously: when recommendations for lifestyle change confront biological adaptations," *The Lancet, Diabetes & Endocrinology* 3:4 (April 2015):232—234. Available at
   http://www.thelancet.com/journals/landia/article/PIIS2213-8587(15)00009-1/fulltext (accessed August 25, 2015). I strongly recommend a full read of this article. It's not encouraging news, but you are stronger if facing an unwanted reality than if chasing an impossible dream.

2. C. Ochner, D Barrios, C. Lee, and F. Pi-Sunyer, "Biological mechanisms that promote weight regain following weight loss in obese humans," *Physiology & Behavior* 120 (2013): 106–113.

3. M. Rosenbaum and R. Leibel, "Adaptive thermogenesis in humans," *International Journal of Obesity* 34:1 (October 2010): S47—S55.

4. University of Illinois McKinley Health Center, "Breaking Down Your Metabolism," May 4, 2010,
   http://www.mckinley.illinois.edu/handouts/metabolism.htm (accessed December 31, 2015).

5. S. Roberts and I. Rosenberg, "Nutrition and Aging: Changes in the Regulation of Energy Metabolism with Aging," *Physiological Reviews* 86:2 (April 2006): 651-667. Also available at http://physrev.physiology.org/content/86/2/651 (accessed December 31, 2015).

6. F.S. Luppino, L.M. de Wit, P.F. Bouvy, T. Stignen, P. Cuijpers, B.W. Penninx, and F.G. Zitman, "Overweight, obesity, and depression: a

Chapter 18 (continued)

systematic review and meta-analysis of longitudinal studies," *Archives of General Psychiatry*, 67:3 (March 2010): 220-229.

7. CDC, "Losing Weight," May 15, 2015, http://www.cdc.gov/healthyweight/losing_weight (accessed May 27, 2016).
8. It is vital to keep weight loss within healthy limits because overeaters occasionally swing to the other extreme and become overly restrictive about their eating. This is just a different way to have an unhealthy relationship with food, creating a different set of serious health risks.

Chapter 20—Daring to be Different

1. This assessment should not be done by a physician associated with a commercially marketed weight loss program, due to inherent conflicts of interest. Your best bet is a physician whom you already know and trust, who has nothing but your best interests to consider.

Chapter 22—Our Need for Reward: The Key to It All

1. External rewards are also sometimes referred to as extrinsic rewards. The terms have the same meaning.
2. Internal rewards are also sometimes referred to as intrinsic rewards. The terms have the same meaning.

Chapter 23—Using Rewards to Drive Results

1. Terry Orlick, *Embracing Your Potential* (Champaign, IL: Human Kinetics, 1998).
2. K.R. Sparrow, *Resiliency and Vulnerability in Girls During Cognitively Challenging Tasks*, Pd.D. dissertation, Florida State University, Tallahassee (1998).

Chapter 24—Dealing with Unwanted Feelings and Bad Days

1. Positive emotions are also a trigger for overeating in many people, but are not the focus of this chapter. Positive emotions are high-energy states, so if you're looking for a non-food alternative for expressing them, consider high-energy options that involve some sort of physical movement. For example, try something like a walk on a pretty day while you bask in the glow of whatever has gotten you into such a good mood.
2. William T. Harbaugh, Ulrich Mayr, and Daniel R. Burghart, "Neural Responses to Taxation and Voluntary Giving Reveal Motives for

Chapter 24 (continued)

Charitable Donations," *Science* 5831:316 (June 15, 2007): 1622-1625. Additional commentary referencing this research is available at http://pages.uoregon.edu/thinking/altruism.html (accessed February 4, 2016).

3. David Burns, *Feeling Good: The New Mood Therapy*, (New York, NY: Harper, 2008).

Chapter 25—Taking Care of Yourself When You Least Feel Like It

1. Nick Hall, *Preventing and Managing Chronic Inflammation, Special Focus: Nutritional Interventions*, (Los Banos, CA: Institute for Brain Potential, 2015). This is a continuing education course for professionals, available on CDs or DVDs purchased directly from the Institute for Brain Potential.

Chapter 26—Thinking More Effectively About Food

1. A handy way to clarify this is to remember that, for example, a tomato is food, while a snack cake is not food. There are many things we can eat that are hard to categorize clearly, however, because they are made of multiple ingredients, only some of which are real food. In those cases, you might consider more generalized terms like *mostly food*, or *mostly not food*, with the understanding that it's not a good sign if it's that hard to tell. Another litmus test is to consider whether, if you made the mystery food a major component of your diet, you would be likely to become more or less healthy as a result.

Chapter 27—Planning for Long-Term Success

1. It's a great idea, once you've identified some canned items and cereals that meet your requirements, to buy them in bulk when they're on sale and then always to replenish your supply well before you actually run out.

2. Marlene Busko, "'Food Desert' Dwellers Have Worse Heart-Disease Risk Profiles," *Medscape* (Apr 05, 2016). Available to members at http://www.medscape.com/viewarticle/861501?nlid=103571_3802 #vp_1 (accessed April 16, 2016).

3. Dr. Marion Nestle has written a very helpful book for the purpose of figuring out what to eat and how to sort through the various options that confront you when you shop: *What to Eat*, (New York: North Point Press, 2006).

Chapter 29—Being Part of the Solution: Support of Others

1. J. Reedy and S. Krebs-Smith, "Dietary Sources of Energy, Solid Fats, and Added Sugars among Children and Adolescents in the United States," *Journal of the American Dietetic Association* 110:10 (October 2010): 1477—1484. Available at http://nccor.org/downloads/roundtable/Reedy%20Krebs%20Smith-%20Dietary%20Sources%20of%20Solid%20Fats.pdf (accessed November 29, 2015).

Chapter 31—Moving as if Your Life Depends on It

1. American College of Sports Medicine, National Exercise Trainer Association, and Aerobics and Fitness Association of America.
2. CDC, "How much physical activity do adults need?" June 4, 2015, http://www.cdc.gov/physicalactivity/basics/adults (accessed April 7, 2016).
3. The National Weight Control Registry, "NWCR Facts," http://www.nwcr.ws/research (accessed April 7, 2016).

Chapter 32—Eating to Live

1. *Merriam-Webster's Collegiate Dictionary, 11ᵗʰ edition*, (Springfield, MA: Meriam-Webster, Inc., 2006): 594.
2. Nick Hall, *Preventing and Managing Chronic Inflammation, Special Focus: Nutritional Interventions*, (Los Banos, CA: Institute for Brain Potential, 2015). This is a continuing education course for professionals, available on CDs or DVDs purchased directly from the Institute for Brain Potential.
3. Special thanks to Katherine Stephens-Bogard, MS, RDN/LD, CDE, RYT for valuable additions to this section, as well as for helpful perspectives that improved the text elsewhere.
4. B. Wansink and J. Sobal, "Mindless Eating: The 200 Daily Food Decisions We Overlook," *Environment and Behavior* 39:1 (2007): 106-123.
5. Brian Wansink, *Mindless Eating* (New York: Bantam, 2006): 65—68.
6. Ibid., 58—60.

Chapter 33—Keeping It Together in Challenging Situations

1. Though I have not done it myself, I have it on good authority that you can successfully microwave plain popcorn with no added oils. The recommendation is to put about 1/4 cup of popcorn kernels

Chapter 33 (continued)
into a paper lunch bag, and then microwave it for two to three minutes. When the rate of popping slows to one time every second or two, you're done.

Chapter 34—Pros and Cons of Some Familiar Strategies
1. Compulsive Eaters Anonymous HOW, http://www.ceahow.org.

Appendix B—Considerations for Restaurant Buffets
1. Brian Wansink, *Mindless Eating* (New York: Bantam, 2006): 65–68.
2. Brian Wansink, *Mindless Eating* (New York: Bantam, 2006): 70-75.

Appendix D—Considerations and Strategies for Hosting Special Meals
1. Brian Wansink, *Mindless Eating* (New York: Bantam, 2006): 70-75.

Appendix F—A Word About Bulimia
1. Mayo Clinic, "Diseases and Conditions—Bulimia nervosa," http://www.mayoclinic.org/diseases-conditions/bulimia/home/ovc-20179821 (accessed May 3, 2016).

Recommended Reading

The books in this list are not the only good ones out there, but they are books that I know well and believe to be exceptional. I have recommended each of them many, many times. Each will support your efforts in a unique and valuable way.

The End of Overeating, by David Kessler (New York, NY: Rodale, Inc., 2009).

Written by a former overeater who was also the FDA Commissioner for eight years, this book is a brilliant exposé of how the food industry purposely engineers its products to be addictive. Once you see this described in detail, you will understand why certain edible products (calling them food is an overstatement) are so likely to result in loss of control. I consider this a must-read for anyone with overeating issues.

Feeling Good: The New Mood Therapy, by David Burns (New York, NY: Harper, 2008).

The author will help you explore the role that internal self-talk has in determining your moods, sense of self, and overall quality of life. You will learn how to identify distorted thinking (we all have some), catch yourself in the act of doing it, and then redirect yourself to more fact-based, empowering alternatives. You will be amazed at how much better this work can help you feel.

Food Rules, by Michael Pollan (New York, NY: Penguin Books, 2009).

This is a simple, clear set of helpful guidelines to use when choosing and consuming food. It's a short, easy read because remember, proper nutrition isn't hard.

Forks Over Knives, by T. Colin Campbell and Caldwell B. Esselstyn (New York, NY: The Experiment, LLC, 2011).

This book (a companion to the excellent DVD of the same title) offers compelling research to suggest that the vegetarian lifestyle can prevent or reverse many serious health conditions. The idea is that you manage your health with your fork rather than with a surgeon's knife. Whether or not you are interested in more vegetarian living, the research and recipes are well worth having.

Going Home, by Gregory Boothroyd and Lori Boothroyd (Delton, MI: Greenwood Associates, 2005).

We all have patterns that we repeat despite the fact that they predictably complicate our lives as we get in our own way. We may even see this and know better, yet feel compelled to keep doing it anyway. This wonderful little book will guide you through the process of deconstructing any such pattern that is keeping you stuck, and then rebuilding something better in its place.

Happier, by Tal Ben-Shahar (New York, NY: McGraw-Hill, 2007).

You probably already know a great deal about what makes you happier than food ever can, but chances are you don't use that knowledge very actively in how you structure your life. This book will help you to discover (or remember) what really brings satisfaction to your life, so you can prioritize accordingly. You'll miss the most important lessons here if you just read it without doing the thought and written exercises that the author suggests—I promise you they are worth the extra time.

How to Cook Everything: The Basics, by Mark Bittman (Hoboken, NJ: Double B Publishing, 2012).

This book is perfect for anyone who avoids cooking because they feel like they don't know what they're doing. The author is clear and easy to follow as he explains everything the beginning home cook needs to know.

He starts with what you need in terms of utensils and cookware to set up your kitchen, then discusses in detail the basic seasonings and staple items you'll want to keep on hand so that you'll always be in a good position to "whip something up" when you need to. He discusses all of the various foods on which you'll base your cooking—pasta, grains, vegetables, beans, meat, poultry, and seafood—preparing you for what it will be like to work with each one and providing lots of handy tips for bringing out their best as you cook.

There are many recipes, all with detailed instructions and photographs which show you exactly what to expect and how to handle each phase of a recipe as you prepare it. This book is the next best thing to having a friendly professional chef helping you figure things out right in your own kitchen. It covers everything from boiling water (really) to putting together a menu for entertaining guests.

The emphasis of this book is *not* low-calorie cooking, just to be clear. However, it is an indispensable resource if low confidence is what's keeping you out of the kitchen.

In Defense of Food, by Michael Pollan (New York, NY: Penguin Press, 2008).

Many of us have forgotten what real food is and why it is important to keep it in our lives despite the availability of cheap, highly processed alternatives. This book will help you find your way back to food that is the foundation of a truly fulfilling life.

Mindless Eating: Why We Eat More Than We Think, by Brian Wansink (New York, NY: Bantam Books, 2006).

This is a brilliant and entertaining look into the psychological quirks and environmental cues that trigger us to eat more or less, and to choose the foods that we do. You can use this information to make simple tweaks to your own life, automatically reducing the amount that you eat without even noticing the difference or feeling deprived. As the author says, "The best diet is the one you don't know you're on."

What to Eat, by Marion Nestle (New York, NY: North Point Press, 2006).

The author is a nationally known nutritionist who has written extensively for the purpose of educating the public. This excellent work, very aptly titled, is a walk through each section of your grocery store, detailing what you will see, what it all means, and how best to choose.

Younger Next Year, and **Younger Next Year for Women,** by Chris Crowley and Henry S. Lodge (New York, NY: Workman Publishing Company, Inc., 2005).

These wonderful books are directed toward people in their fifties and beyond, but are highly advisable for anyone in adulthood. This information is best used sooner rather than later, but later is *far* better than not at all. It is a broad-brush approach to creating your highest quality of life, with heavy emphasis on maximizing your physical health, the necessary platform for all else. The material is informative and motivating; it's an easy and entertaining read.

8 Steps to a Pain-Free Back, by Esther Gokhale (Stanford, CA: Pendo Press, 2008).

This excellent book may seem like an odd addition to this particular reading list, which is why I placed it last, but I included it for a very specific reason. It explains our epidemic of back pain as the result of our way of life being very different from that to which we're adapted, a theme that you may now recognize more clearly. It reinforces the lesson that the best life is possible only when we live in alignment with our bodies' needs.

If you use the teachings of this book to reduce your back pain, you will accomplish two valuable things. First, your emotional brain will be a lot calmer because you're not in as much pain. Second, your body will feel better and become capable of a greater range of physical activities, giving you more ways to enjoy your life.

This material is a surprisingly good companion to the work you're doing with food because it shows another facet of connecting with, taking care of, and having a better experience with your body.

About the Author

Elizabeth Babcock, LCSW was a tormented overeater for 37 years but has now maintained comfortable balance with food since 2001. She specializes in psychotherapy with others who overeat, along with conducting community education seminars and trainings for healthcare professionals.

She resides in southwestern Pennsylvania where she spends as much time as possible outdoors when weather permits, preferably walking, kayaking, or lazing in a hammock with a good book. She can be reached at www.elizabethbabcock.com and on Facebook.

Made in the USA
Lexington, KY
05 January 2018